THE
Cannabis Gardener

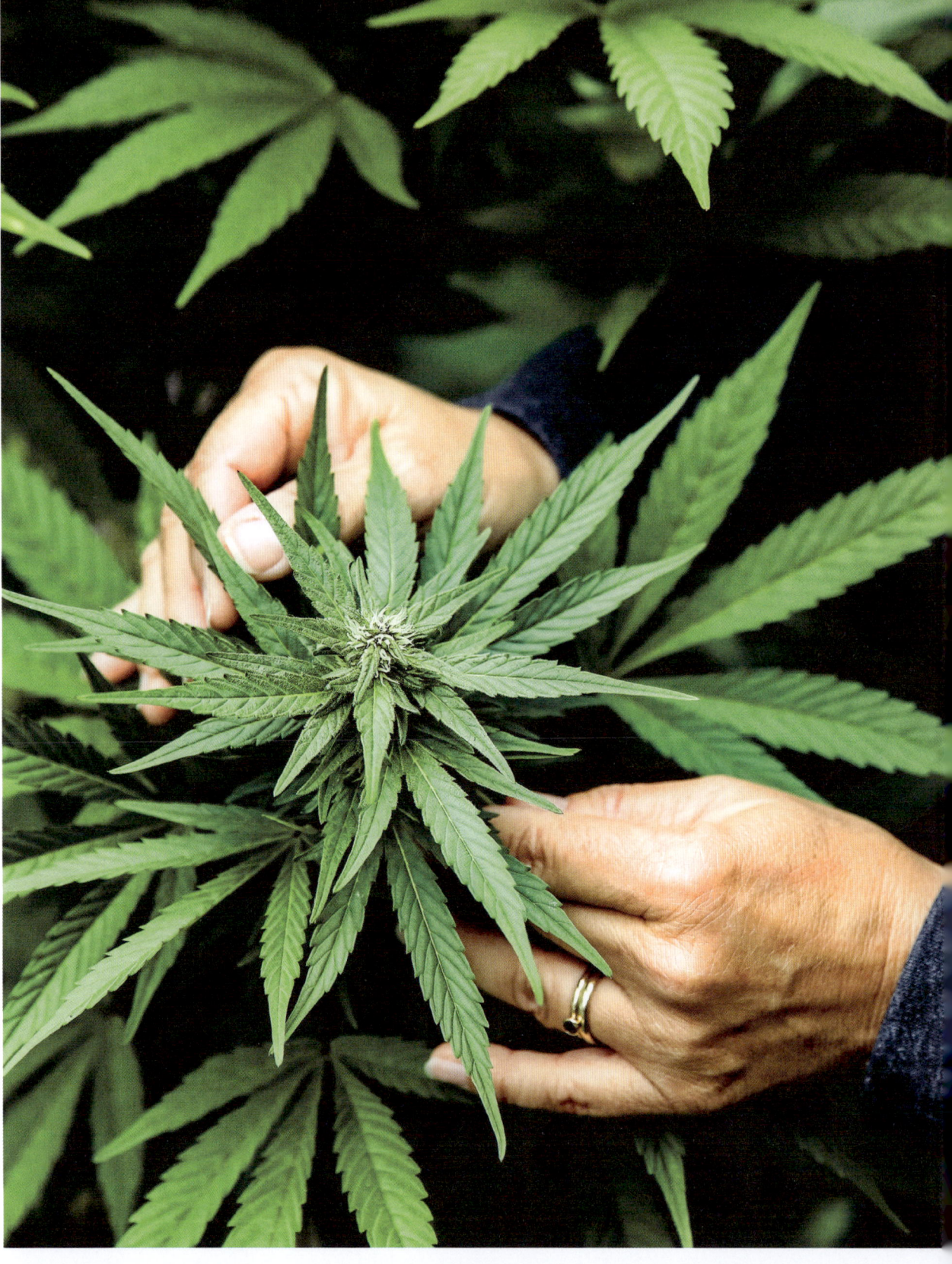

THE Cannabis Gardener

A beginner's guide to growing vibrant,
healthy plants in every region

PENNY BARTHEL
Photography by Erin Scott

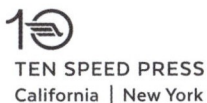
TEN SPEED PRESS
California | New York

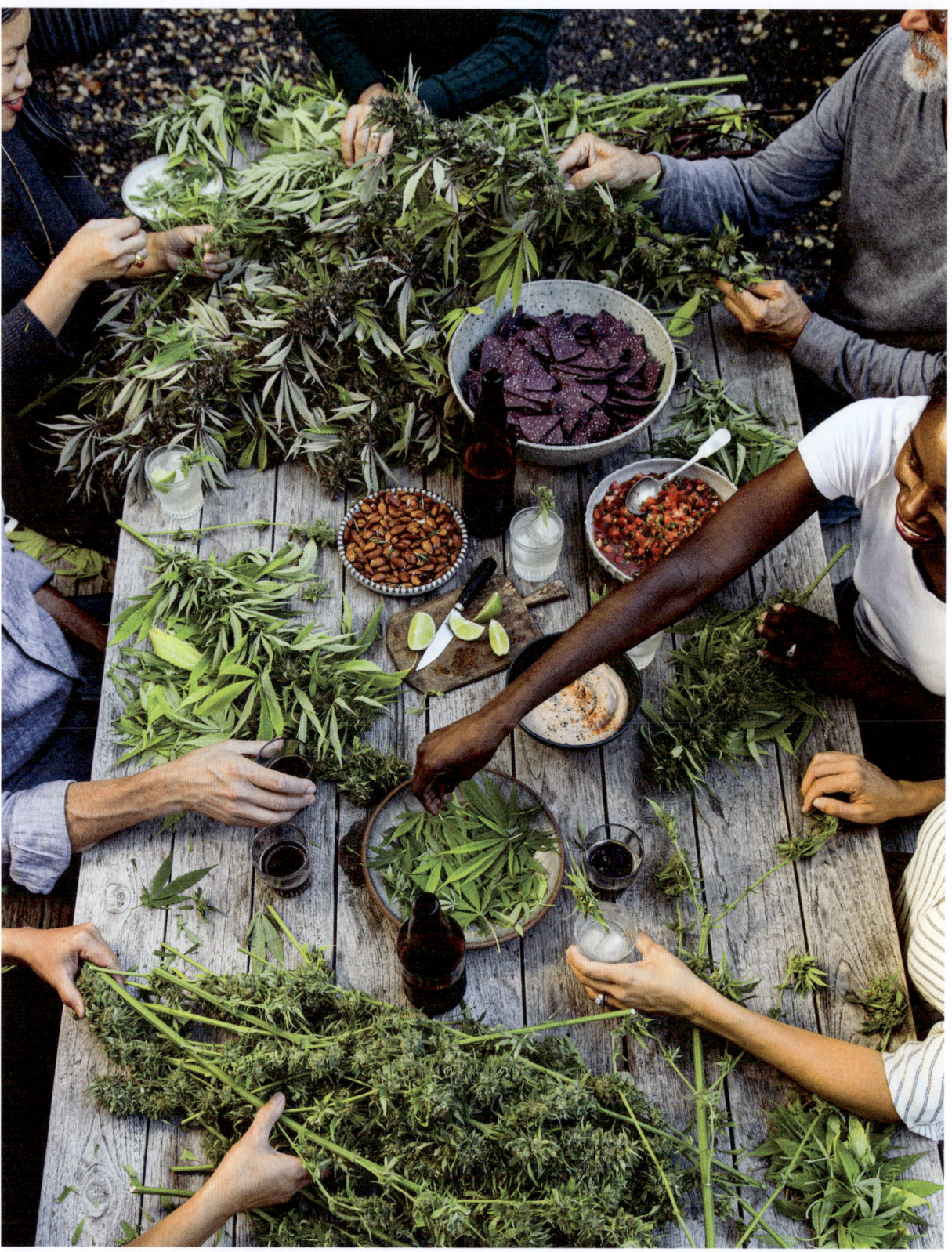

Contents

Introduction

Cannabis is one of humanity's most useful plants. It is also one of the most notorious and misunderstood plants of all time. It is at once a durable fiber, nourishing food, a health aid, a euphoriant, a social lubricant. It is also—according to US federal law—a schedule 1 drug, meaning that it is considered to be a substance of the highest danger and lowest value to humanity. Is cannabis really all of these things at once? Yes, it is. But we are in a new era, both in the United States and globally.

State by state, cannabis is being legalized, and the pressure is building to de-schedule this gift of nature and create a sane and wholesome appreciation for the potential that this plant can bring to the world. And best of all? It's really fun to grow in the garden. With a planter, some soil, a cannabis seed, and a spot in the sun, anyone can grow healthy cannabis. I believe that everyone should have access to the gifts of physical, emotional, and spiritual health that cannabis offers to humanity.

I live in California, where cannabis possession and consumption is legal statewide and cultivation is broadly permitted for personal use. Cannabis regulation is constantly changing, making it important for citizens to stay up to date with the latest information. (NORML.org is an excellent resource for remaining informed.) This recent freedom for weed enthusiasts is not by chance, though. It is the outcome of many hard-won victories by cannabis growers and activists. We owe a debt to people like Dennis Peron and Mary Jane Rathbun, who fought and sacrificed to bring this healing plant out of the prohibition era and into the legal post–prohibition era. Northern California has been the literal seedbed of cannabis innovation and hybridization for the past several decades. I am so grateful for the work of the cannabis warriors who paid dearly for my gardening freedom. But there is still work to be done. Let's be clear: The war on drugs is rooted in racism and white supremacy. Too many people linger in prison from minor cannabis convictions, and these people are disproportionately people of color. Even after they have served their time, their convictions linger over them, making it difficult to obtain employment or regain the right to vote. I encourage each of us to put our voices and votes toward record expungement and cannabis de-scheduling and legalization on a national level. Let's all support our local BIPOC and equity cannabis businesses and give those who've paid an unfair price some space to grow in the new cannabis economy.

To celebrate the new post–prohibition era, consider planting your own cannabis victory garden. There is so much great weed to enjoy, grow, and learn from. Its resins contain unique molecules that are active in just about every cell in the human body—indeed in every mammal's body. Thankfully, cannabis is an undemanding plant in the garden. It grows just about anywhere and completes its entire life in under a year. The cannabis gardener is free to explore the abundance that this plant offers without the constraints of needing to turn a profit—that's the work of the cannabis farmer. We gardeners have freedom to experiment with different cultivars and growing techniques because we're our own clients. We can make mistakes without the fear of financial ruin. I think the best part of growing my own weed is how much joy it brings me. From a small green-gray seed firmly rooted in my own soil comes a magnificent 10-foot-tall beauty, covered with richly scented, sparkly flower buds. And from these flower buds, sticky with resins, I get to craft tinctures, salves, and edibles that keep me feeling great throughout the year. I invite you to join me in an adventure of connection and become a cannabis gardener.

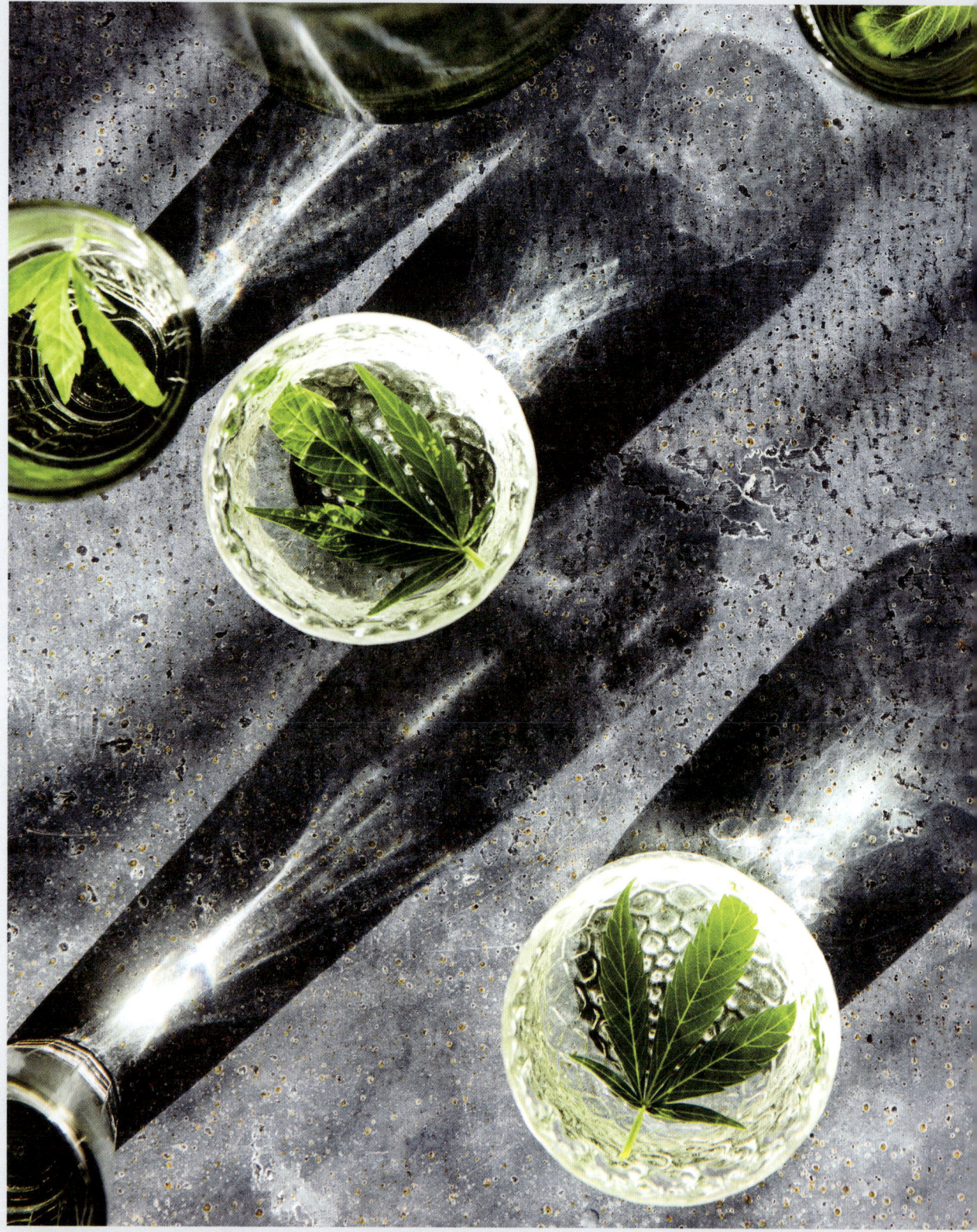

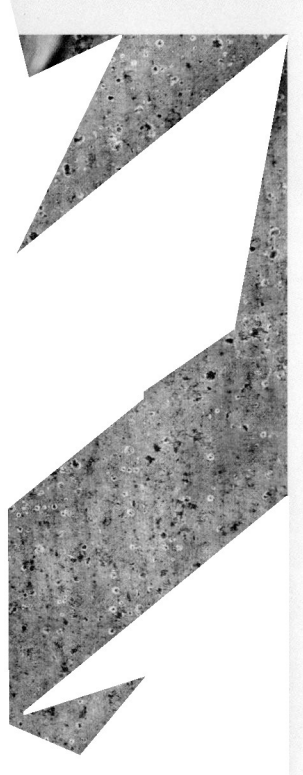

CHAPTER 1

Choosing the Right Cannabis for You and Your Garden

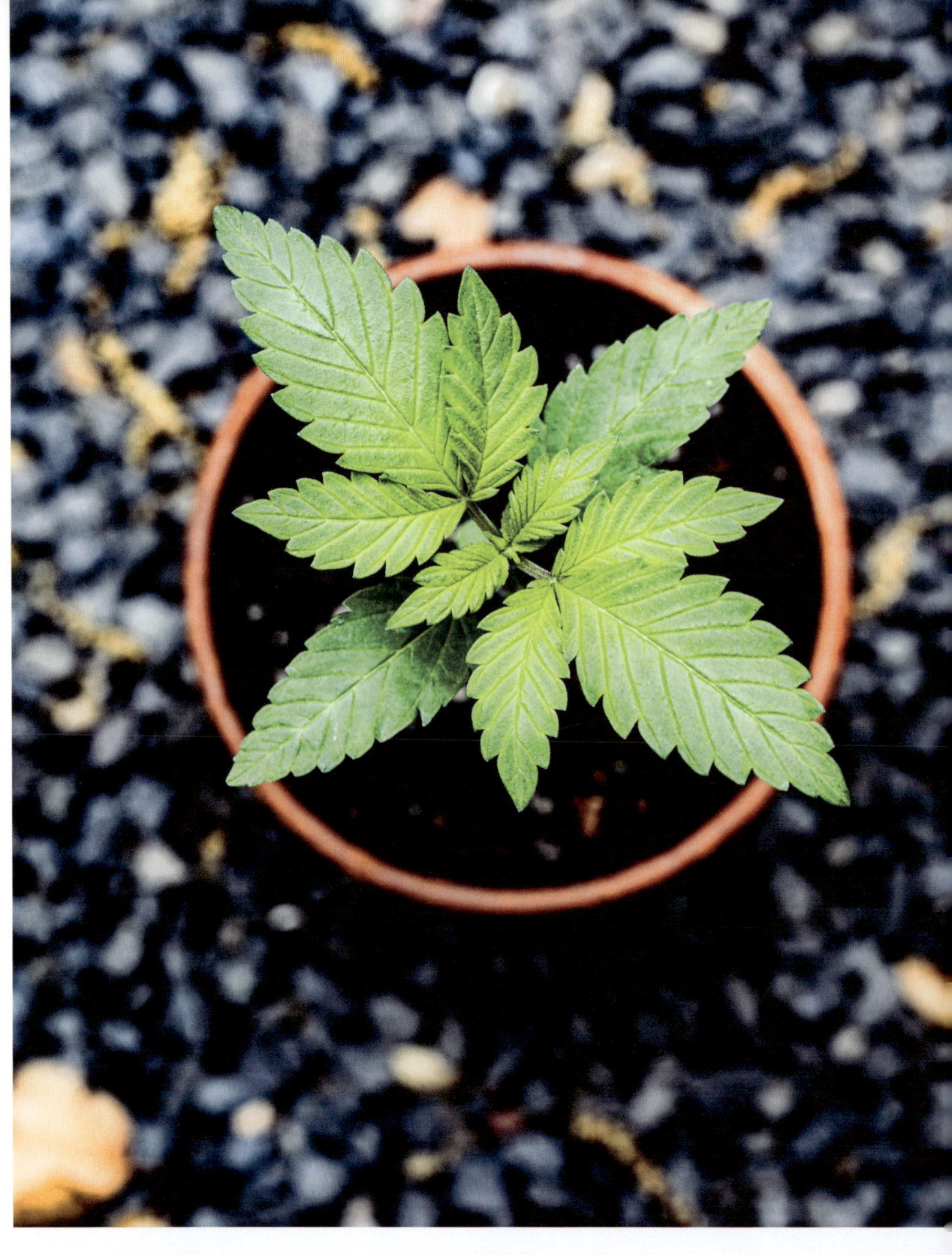

> Cannabis is one of the world's most useful plant groups. It has been a part of human culture for thousands of years beginning in Eurasia, and today it is associated with people in almost all parts of the world.
>
> —ROBERT C. CLARKE AND MARK D. MERLIN, *Cannabis Evolution and Ethnobotany*

CANNABIS— THE PLANT

Growing up in suburban California, I first heard about cannabis while I was in junior high. Televised antidrug ads blasted, "This is your brain. This is your brain on drugs," while showing an egg frying in a hot pan (and that image will forever linger in my psyche). Cheech and Chong provided my main information on cannabis, since I was raised smack-dab in the middle of the war on drugs. Currently the word *weed* has surfaced, and I've also heard it called many different names, some of them reflective of the form that the harvested plant product takes, such as, hashish. Other names come from local slang, such as pakalōlō in Hawaii. Ganja, grass, maryjane, doobie—there are all sorts of slang terms for cannabis and the things made from it. Some of these terms are enduring and ancient; others have popped up quite recently.

While this plant has many nicknames, its commonly used scientific name is *Cannabis sativa*—for now, at least. The influential Swedish taxonomist Carolus Linnaeus provided this name for the scientific community in his book *Species Plantarum* in 1753. Like many botanical names, the name *Cannabis sativa* has been bandied about by the scientific community for hundreds of years. As an understanding of plant origins changes, scientists sometimes radically adjust how to classify, and thus name, particular plants. Cannabis has at different times been classified as one, two, or three separate species. You may have heard the terms *indica* and *sativa* offered as different species of cannabis. These same two terms are used in another way: to describe certain effects by type of cannabis. A third group, *ruderalis,* is well known to cannabis breeders—especially those interested in breeding auto-flowering plants.

I think it's quite illuminating that we use the name *sativa* for the species name of this plant. The term *sativa* in botanical nomenclature refers to any useful, health-promoting cultivated plant—precisely what cannabis is. For this book, I will use the terms *cannabis* and *weed* interchangeably. But whichever name is used, I believe cannabis is a plant of *connection*. It helps us connect to ourselves, to each other, and to the natural world. Cannabis gardeners have the special joy of being invited into the whole life of this plant while being outside, in the sun, and part of a natural process.

THE HUMAN HISTORY OF CANNABIS

People have used cannabis for a very long time—for fiber, food, medicine, and mood enhancement. Cannabis has also been used in religious rituals for at least twenty-five thousand years and has been cultivated commercially for six thousand years. While cannabis does grow in the wild, it is difficult to separate the truly wild-type cannabis groups from those that humans have influenced. Researchers aren't even sure of what cannabis was first used for. It may have been for fiber, spiritual use, or for the mood-enhancing qualities of inhaled smoke. What we do know is that people have enjoyed and benefitted from cannabis for millennia.

Cannabis likely originated in the wild in central Asia. This ancient plant grew best in areas with abundant sunshine, nitrogen-rich soil, consistent summer moisture, and pronounced seasonal daylight changes. Interestingly, cannabis grows really well in conditions also attractive to humans—near bodies of freshwater with rich soil. As soon as people discovered cannabis, they began changing it to suit their needs. And the cannabis plant responded generously to those demands. Cannabis is quite plastic in its ability to adapt to selective breeding. That is why some varieties of the plant grow stick straight and tall, with long fibrous stalks, while others grow short and dense with richly scented, sticky flowers.

As people ventured to other lands, they brought cannabis seeds with them. Cannabis seeds don't spread easily by themselves, but when humans figured out how useful this plant was, they gathered the seeds of their favorite plants to grow when they moved to a new place. Cannabis adapted to new climates easily, creating stable breeding populations with unique characteristics. Some cultures favored certain uses for the cannabis plant. Japan and Korea prized cannabis as a fiber for cloth, selecting cannabis that grew lanky with long leaf internodes (areas of stem between leaves). Other groups used cannabis as medicine and chose plants fragrant with sticky resin. During the age of expansion, as traders moved across vast oceans, they, too, brought cannabis to new lands. As a result, we find

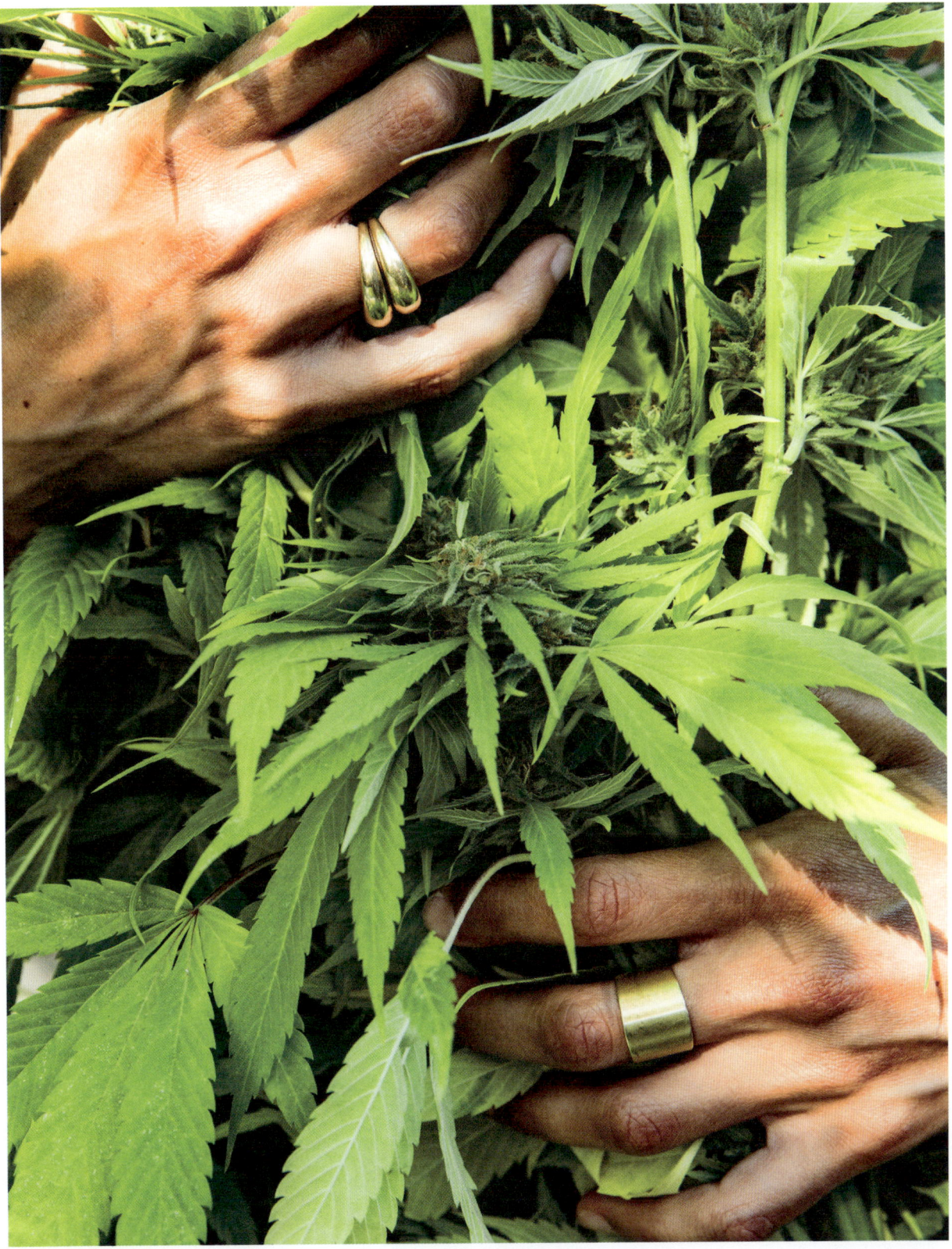

stable cannabis populations with widely varied traits in different areas around the globe. Known as landraces, these plants aren't wild, since they were originally distributed by people, but they are better understood as being feral plants. Some famous landraces are Hindu Kush from the Afghan/Pakistan region, Acapulco Gold from Mexico, Durban Poison from Africa, Thai from Southeast Asia, and Colombian Gold from Central America. If you hear someone telling you they are growing true wild-type weed, it's likely not true. That's not to say that their cannabis isn't amazing; it's just that cannabis is so adaptable to human influence that it's a challenge to keep a population truly wild and unaffected by people.

Landraces are stable, naturally growing cannabis that populate different places in the world. They are a product of human influence, but grow on their own in nature. They are rather like the wild parrots of Telegraph Hill in San Francisco, but even more regionalized.

Today, cannabis is commercially cultivated for resin-rich flowers, seed for food and oil, fiber for cloth and rope, animal bedding, eyeglasses, car parts, building foundation materials such as hempcrete, and fuel such as hemp biodiesel. This is one versatile and helpful plant!

CHOOSING WHICH PLANT TO GROW

Before you plant your first cannabis, there are two big decisions to make. The first question to ask yourself is "What do I want from my cannabis harvest?" The second question is "What cannabis cultivars will grow well in my garden?" Let's explore these two questions.

What do I want from my cannabis harvest? Why am I growing this plant? I ask you to pause and consider your hopes for your grow—because this will be key information as you seek out the best cannabis match for you. A wide variety of cannabis seeds and clones are available to the home grower—and there's more variety available with each passing year. And as recent discoveries unlock some of the mystery of this plant, the way to choose what cannabis to grow is changing dramatically. Rather than relying on anecdotal evidence about the potency and impact of a cultivar, today's growers have access to concrete biochemical information to guide their choices.

As you think first about what you want from your grow, take a minute to jot down some of your hopes. Perhaps you're looking for some awesome dank bud to enjoy at the end of the day—and are after a huge sparkly cola. Maybe you're interested in managing the pain of arthritis. If you're

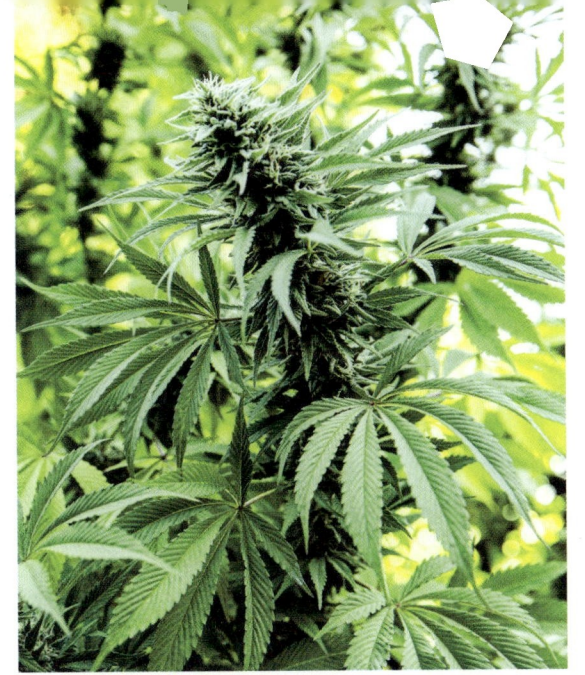

a curious gardener, like me, then it could be that you're always on the hunt for a cool new plant to try in your soil. One of the reasons a friend of mine grew her first cannabis plant was to support a friend of hers who was battling cancer and benefitted from smoking weed but couldn't afford to buy much at the dispensary. (Plus—let's be honest—she wanted some for herself.) Whatever your reasons, know that cannabis is an expressive plant and offers us humans a wide array of benefits: health support, mood enhancement, and lush beauty for the garden.

One of the reasons I grow cannabis is to support my health. I—like many people—get aches and pains from working out, have emerging osteoarthritis, occasional migraines, and am a sensitive sleeper. Oh—and I have reactive skin and rosacea, too. Guess what? Cannabis is helpful for all those things. Being an inquisitive person, I like to go deep when I learn, so I wondered about how cannabis could help with this wide array of issues. Frankly, I was a little skeptical when I overheard conversations or read about the extraordinary claims being made about the helpfulness of cannabis for human health. I wondered how one plant could provide relief for such a wide variety of health problems. It was tempting to shut my mind to the claims, but I resisted the temptation and decided to dig in instead. What a good decision that was and continues to be. Hang on, dear reader—there is a large and important body of studies emerging, and that is very good news for us all. The way cannabis works in the body is both fascinating and hope giving. My own understanding of the science has also increased my confidence in selecting cannabis to improve my health and well-being. Throughout this book, I'll share some of what I've learned about how cannabis impacts human health and offer guidance to help you make the best cannabis plant match for both your body's and your garden's needs.

THE ENDO-CANNABINOID SYSTEM

We are a part of nature—we all know this. But our modern human-built environments can sometimes fool us into forgetting our creatureliness. When we grow, cultivate, harvest, and use our own cannabis, we are reminded of our place in the natural world. As we share a joint or offer a friend some of our homemade cannabis tincture, we are connecting to other people. Our collective human experiences inform us that this plant

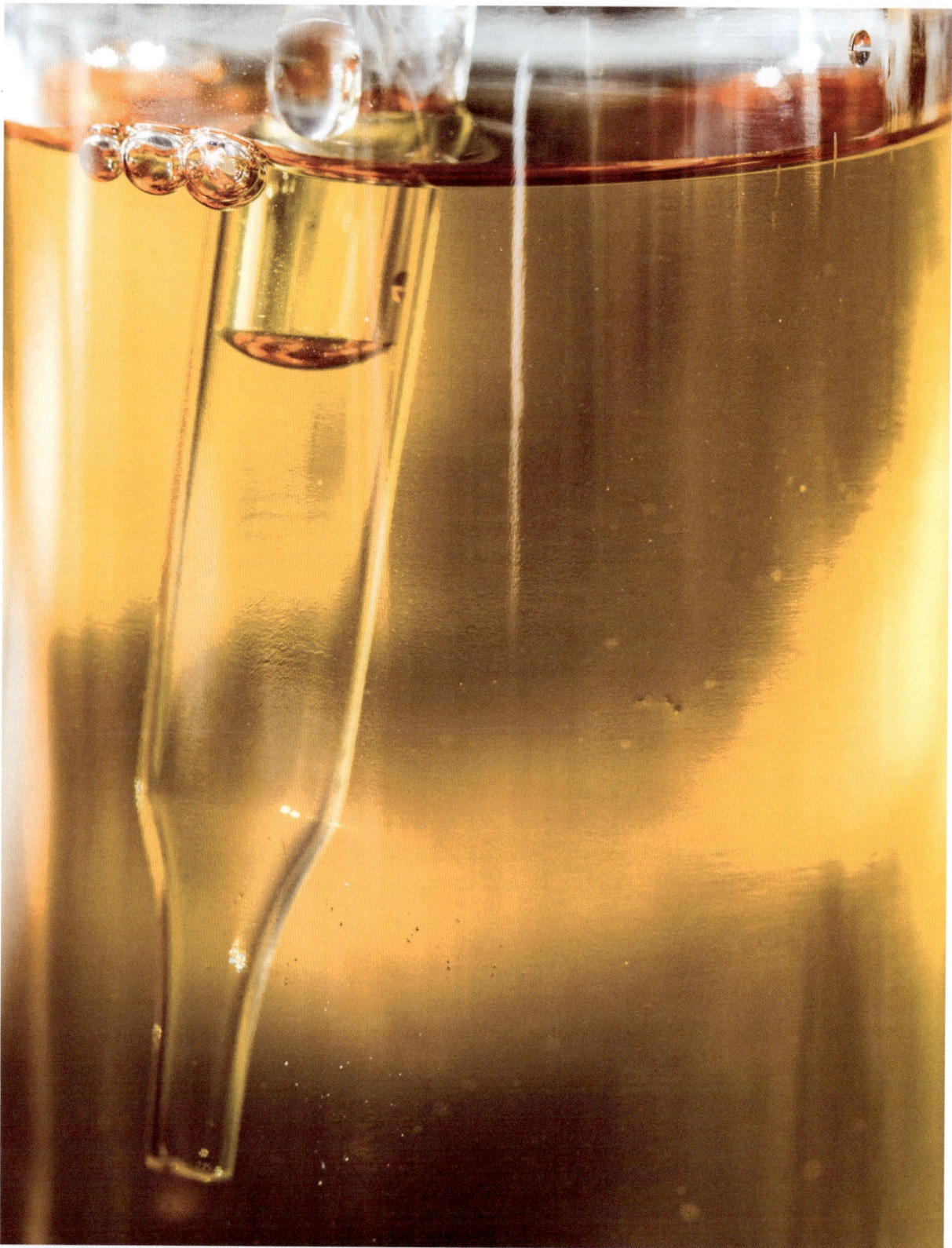

is—and has been for millennia—at work in us for the better. But just how and why cannabis impacts us has been a mystery until rather recently. Today, we are witnessing a new era in cannabis history.

You may be familiar with systems in the human body—including the circulatory, skeletal, lymph, respiratory, nervous, digestive, and muscular systems. You probably learned about these in science class. People have been studying them for hundreds of years. And yet, very recently, a new body system was discovered and named. This system is everywhere in the human body, in all vertebrates—any animal that has a spine—in fact. This system is perhaps the most widely distributed system in our entire body, but until very recently, we knew *nothing* about it. It's called the endocannabinoid system (ECS) and is often referred to as the "bridge between mind and body." We are beginning to understand the ECS as the master system, the one what governs all the other systems. Amazing! Through the discovery of the ECS, we are exploring the ways in which cannabis helps our bodies and minds work better.

First, a little history. In a US government–funded study at the St. Louis University School of Medicine in 1988, two scientists identified receptors for compounds found in cannabis—and they found that these particular types of receptors were more prevalent than *any other* neuroreceptor in the body. This staggeringly significant discovery illuminated a hidden world of activity in the body that has broad significance for our health and well-being. Further studies revealed that there are two endocannabinoid receptors, named CB1 and CB2. Scientists were stunned to learn that CB1 receptors were the single most abundant receptor in the brain. The discovery of the chemicals that affected these two receptors—namely cannabinoids—was a watershed moment for the global scientific community.

A cannabinoid is a substance that affects the ECS. Our bodies make cannabinoids—called endocannabinoids. The two endocannabinoids identified so far are anandamide (AEA), and 2-arachidonoylglycerol (2-AG). Our bodies are in fact constantly making cannabinoids to regulate all sorts of processes to keep us in homeostasis—a balanced state of consistent well-being. Cannabis plants also make cannabinoids—called phytocannabinoids. The cannabis plant isn't making these substances for us but for its own uses. I refer to cannabinoids generally in this book, rather than distinguishing between endocannabinoids and phytocannabinoids. However they come to us, either made in the body or ingested from the cannabis plant, they have a profound impact on our health and mood.

CANNABIS AND HUMAN HEALTH

The ECS is the most pervasive system in our bodies, and its function—broadly explained—is to keep the body in a steady state of health. This master system is involved in supporting a wide array of physiological and mental processes, including fertility, pregnancy, appetite, pain sensation, mood, and memory. One detail about the ECS that is particularly interesting is that it is vital for the proper, healthy functioning of our immune system.

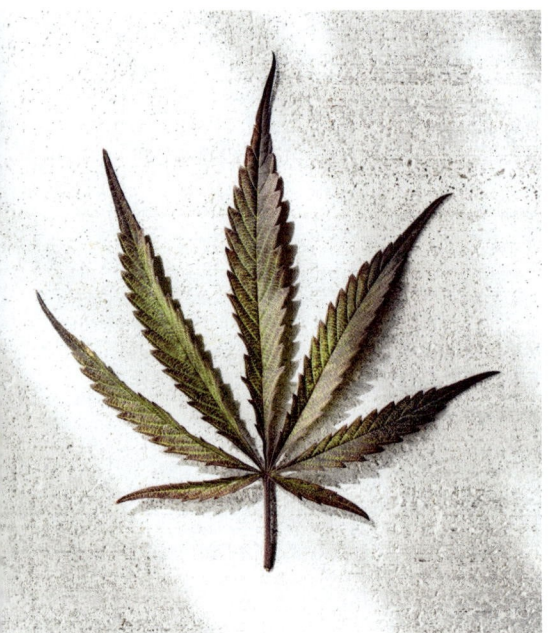

Current cannabis medical research is exciting and helpful for the future of human disease treatment and prevention. In a landmark 2013 National Institutes of Health study entitled "Modulating the Endocannabinoid System in Human Health and Disease," Drs. Pál Pacher and George Kunos stated that "modulating ECS activity may have therapeutic potential in almost all diseases affecting humans." According to this study, almost *all* human diseases are impacted by the ECS, and the cannabinoids and terpenes found in cannabis directly support the ECS. Putting this together, cannabis use may have an impact on nearly all diseases affecting humans. This sweeping statement offers support for the importance of cannabis in human health. Along with its newfound health benefits and its place in safe recreational use, it is ever more appealing for gardeners to grow their own weed and feel better about consuming it.

Growing up in the United States and being educated in public schools have made me a typical post-enlightenment, individualistic, science-trusting person. I have a strong inclination toward Western medicine, both because it's powerful and because this is the culture in which I was raised. And yet, I recognize that it has significant blind spots. Western medicine is great at treating disease but less interested in health support. Our doctors encourage us to be vaccinated, eat good food, and get some exercise, but they often don't suggest much else regarding disease prevention. This leaves an opening for other medicine traditions, including herbal medicine and cannabis that gently and safely offer support to our health. And while we are only at the beginning of understanding how and why cannabinoids impact our lives, we have literally thousands of years' worth of anecdotal evidence to support the safety, relief, and pleasure that this plant brings us.

So, how does this new understanding of the ECS help guide which cannabis plant will be best for our bodies? It helps us figure out which cannabinoids will most likely support our health goals; this in turn will narrow our choice of cultivars. Let's take a look at cannabinoids, terpenes, and the entourage effect.

Cannabinoids

Cannabinoids are a large group of natural compounds made by your body (endocannabinoids) and also made by the cannabis plant (phytocannabinoids). They interact in complex ways with specific receptors in the body and brain, either switching them on or off or momentarily changing the way the receptors work. They work gently, offering support to the body's natural health maintenance. While a cannabis plant manufactures hundreds of cannabinoids, most are found only in tiny amounts. It's helpful to have a basic working vocabulary of the major cannabinoids to help guide your choice of cannabis plants and products. The two most common cannabinoids found in cannabis are THC and CBD.

THC. The most famous cannabinoid is THC, or delta-9-tetrahydrocannabinol, which produces strong mood and health effects. THC is the molecule most responsible for the feelings of euphoria—the "high"—that nearly all of us feel when consuming enough cannabis. By volume, THC is the most abundant cannabinoid in weed grown for resin-rich flower buds. THC works as an anti-inflammatory and pain killer, improves appetite, and has potent psychotropic effects. Taken in large quantity, THC can cause a powerful, sometimes unsettling, psychedelic experience.

While THC is active in both the CB1 and CB2 receptors, its influence on CB1 receptors is of the most interest to patients and recreational users alike. CB1 receptors are abundant in the brain and central nervous system. One part of the brain where there are no CB1 receptors is in the brain stem, the part of the brain responsible for respiration and circulation. This is primary reason why cannabis overdoses do not cause death. For some folks, THC acts to calm racing thoughts, relaxing the mental tension that we occasionally experience. This same reaction can be perceived by some as hypersensitivity to surroundings, or paranoia. Some of us become loquacious, some get sleepy, many get hungry (aka get the "munchies"). And even if we take too much THC (Hit that bong way too hard! Ate the whole brownie!) and have a stronger-than-intended experience, we will recover in several hours to a day. Very few people have ever died directly of cannabis overconsumption. That said, those who are sensitive to psychotropic medicines or who have schizoaffective disorder should be cautious when consuming THC and proceed with tiny doses. A helpful reminder from the medical cannabis community is "low and slow"; keep your dose low and let the impact fully resolve before consuming more. THC starts out as THCa in the cannabis plant. THCa is simply the THC molecule with a small carboxyl group (a carbon atom with two oxygen atoms and one hydrogen atom) attached to it. There is little to no THC in raw, freshly harvested cannabis bud, only THCa.

CBD. The second most abundant cannabinoid is CBD, or cannabidiol. This cannabinoid is everywhere in the news lately—and for good reason. Taken alone, CBD is broadly effective in the body and does not produce intoxicating effects, even at high doses. That doesn't mean it isn't psychoactive—it is! But CBD's effects on the brain, and thus our perception of reality, are mild and non-psychedelic. Most people feel calmed after consuming CBD. CBD also is well established as an anti-seizure medicine and relieves anxiety. It can even be used as a tool to reduce an uncomfortable high if one ingests too much THC. CBD is also anti-inflammatory, anti-microbial, anti-psychotic, and pain-killing—and this is just CBD alone. When CBD gets together with THC and other cannabinoids, its impacts are altered—usually for the better.

CBD is legal in all parts of the United States except Idaho, Iowa, and South Dakota—sold without a prescription in many drugstores and frequently added to cosmetics, coffee, and soft drinks. So why is this particular cannabinoid sold without a prescription in so many places, whereas cannabis flower is still federally a schedule 1 drug? There are a couple of reasons. The first is that CBD can be derived from hemp. Botanically, hemp and cannabis are one and the same. Legally, they are different. The legal definition of hemp is cannabis that contains less than 0.3 percent by dry weight of THC. The 2018 US farm bill made hemp growing legal, and hemp contains enough CBD that commercial isolation of this molecule from the plant has become a big business. But technically speaking, while hemp is legal, concentrated CBD isn't. If you get your CBD from cannabis, it's still illegal! Same molecule, same species, but one is legal, and the other is not. This is the confusing nonsense that will hopefully soon be sorted out by legalizing and de-scheduling this plant.

Other cannabinoids. While you may have heard about THC and CBD before reading this book, you may be less familiar with the hundreds—you heard that right—of other cannabinoids. As we tumble out of prohibition, there has been a burst of activity to study the various cannabinoids found in weed. It seems that every day brings new insights into the different

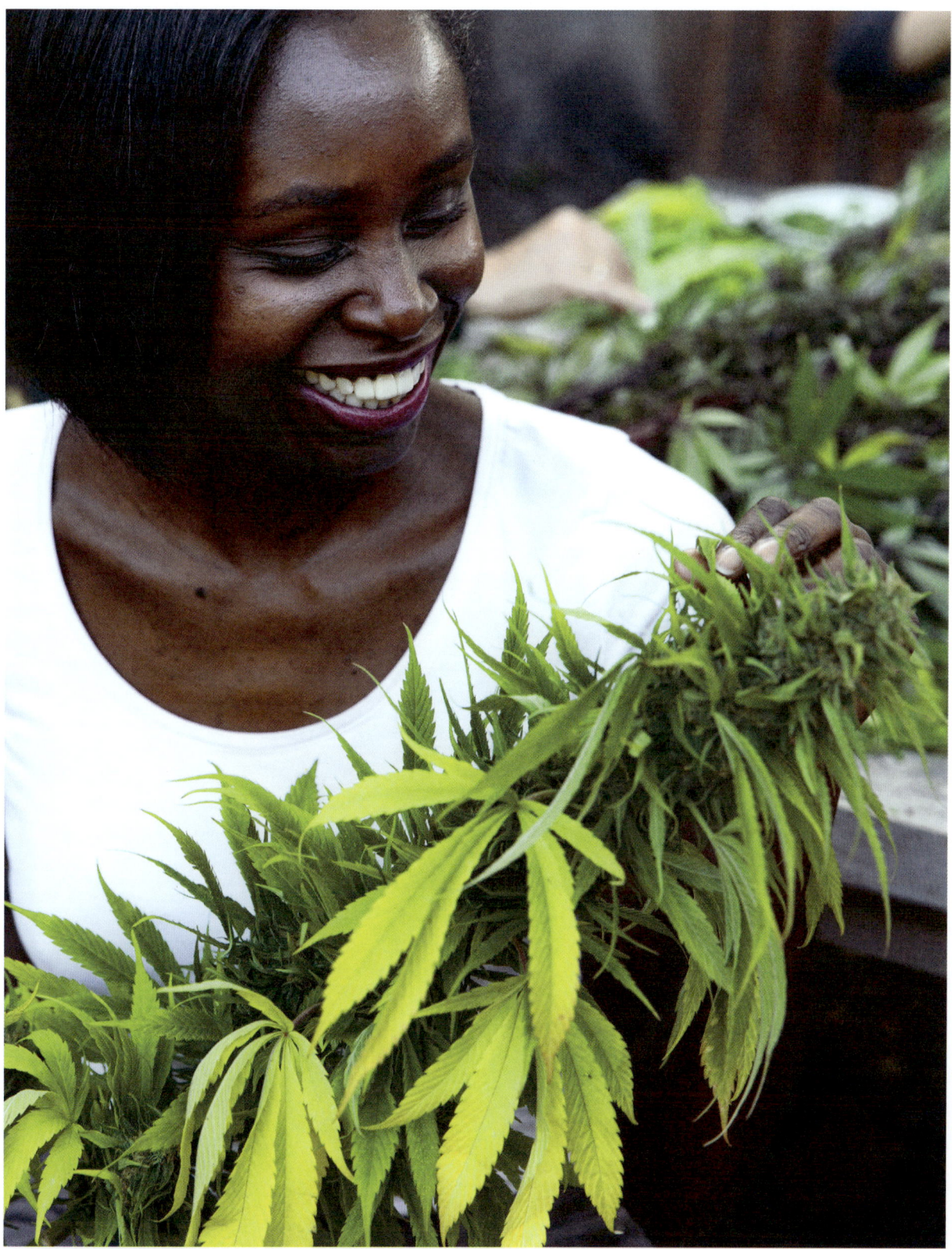

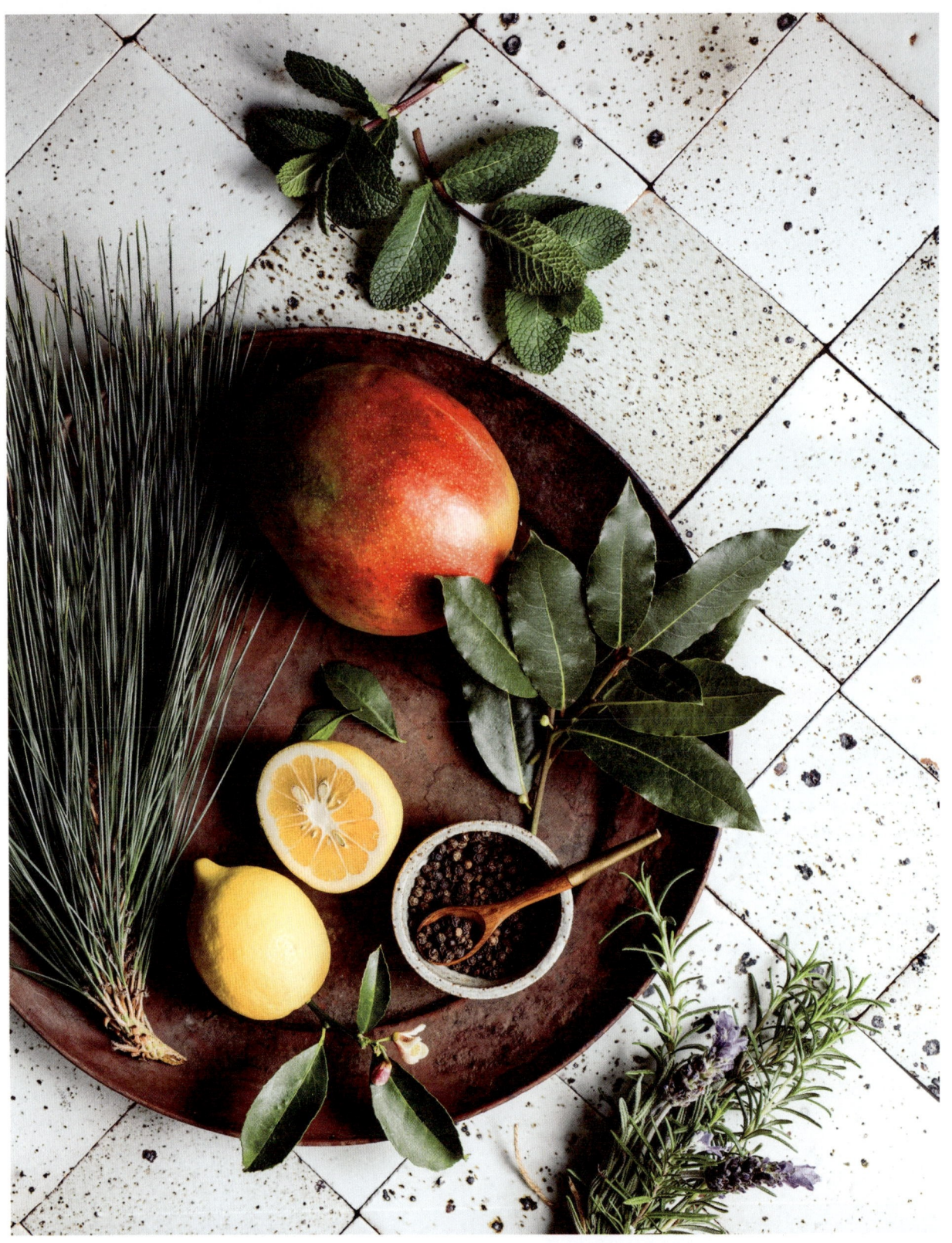

impacts of cannabis on our bodies. Here are a few of the better understood cannabinoids and how they may impact you.

THCa. This is the THC molecule as it's found in the fresh leaf or bud. This cannabinoid is not going to make you high. But it very well may help out with inflammation and pain management. When you whip up a tincture with fresh bud (see page 146), you can access this helpful cannabinoid.

CBDa. This is the CBD molecule as it's found in the fresh leaf or bud. CBDa has been studied for about a decade and is showing promise for treating inflammation—but in a different way entirely from CBD. It's also showing promise as an anti-convulsant.

CBN. Cannabinol, or CBN, is what THCa eventually turns into given enough time. Cannabis flower continues to change slowly after it is harvested: THCa turns into CBNa, which turns into CBN. Heat, light, oxygen, and time are the four most important factors that influence this natural biochemical process. CBN is known for its sedative, soporific effect, which is sometimes referred to as couchlock.

CBG. Cannibigerol, or CBG, is the mother cannabinoid. In the plant, it begins as CBGa and all the other cannabinoids are derived from this one. There is nothing we can do to transform CBG into other cannabinoids— the cannabis plant has to do this. Some breeders are selecting cultivars that retain CBG in their mature flowers, since this cannabinoid is showing medical promise for treating pain, muscle disorders, inflammation, skin disorders, perhaps even depression and cancer. As with most things in the cannabis realm, studies are in progress on CBG. This is an emerging cannabinoid in the supplement market.

CBC. Cannabichromene, or CBC, starts as CBCa in the plant and is a potent, non-intoxicating cannabinoid that has shown the potential to treat pain and inflammation, is neuroprotective, is helpful in treating acne, and may even alleviate depression.

And this is just the tip of the cannabinoid iceberg. There are many cannabinoids found in cannabis preparations, most of them in tiny quantities. Each cultivar of cannabis has its own particular set of cannabinoids and terpenes that interact with each other and our bodies in unique ways.

Terpenes and the Entourage Effect
In addition to cannabinoids, there is another important group of molecules to explore: terpenes. You've experienced terpenes, even if you've never heard this word before, because you can smell them. Whereas

cannabinoids are found primarily in cannabis, terpenes are common in many plants. Cannabis is notoriously fragrant, and terpenes are to blame. Terpenes are important players in how the cannabinoids behave in our bodies. Terpenes are the reason why two cannabis varieties, with nearly identical cannabinoid profiles but varying fragrances or terpene profiles, can affect our bodies differently. This is called the entourage effect, a term coined by Dr. Raphael Mechoulam, who is considered the grandfather of cannabis research. He used the term "entourage effect" to describe the *synergistic effects of cannabinoids and terpenes as they work together in our bodies*. Terpenes impact health, even when used in isolation. When terpenes are consumed with cannabinoids, they interact in our bodies in new ways. Nature has a way of creating symbiosis, and that is true of the hundreds of biologically active molecules found in cannabis.

THE COMPLEXITY OF CANNABIS IN THE BODY

At a recent lecture called "Pleasure, Poison, Prescription, Prayer: The Worlds of Mind-Altering Substances" at the University of California, Berkeley, Dr. David Presti presented "Cannabis Neurobiology: More Complex than Black-Hole Astrophysics." Dr. Presti began his scientific career by studying astrophysics, then switched to molecular biology and biophysics. In his lecture he explained how cannabis works in the brain and body and its relative complexity. To help his audience gain perspective on just how different cannabis is from many other intoxicants, he ticked off a brief explanation of different ones, such as alcohol, caffeine, opium, and nicotine, and their neurologic impacts. For all of these, it was one active molecule and one specific receptor. But when he got to cannabis, the data set changed radically. By contrast, cannabis contains hundreds of distinct molecules that impact receptors found abundantly in the body. Dr. Presti made the bold claim that while he believes future researchers will uncover some of the ways in which cannabis works in the body, we will never know the whole story—it's just too complex, calling it "non-computable," or too complex to fully compute. This is a challenging story to our Western, reductionist mindset for sure. He offered a final thought—a closing benediction. He encouraged us to "just get to know this plant." In other words, don't let the enormous complexity of cannabis's impact on the body be a stumbling block to experimentation.

Let's make some sense of this complexity and narrow in on some good choices for your body. Start by asking yourself, "What do I want from my cannabis harvest?" "Why am I growing this plant?" For many of us, we're looking for a particular impact, often due to health issues. New weed

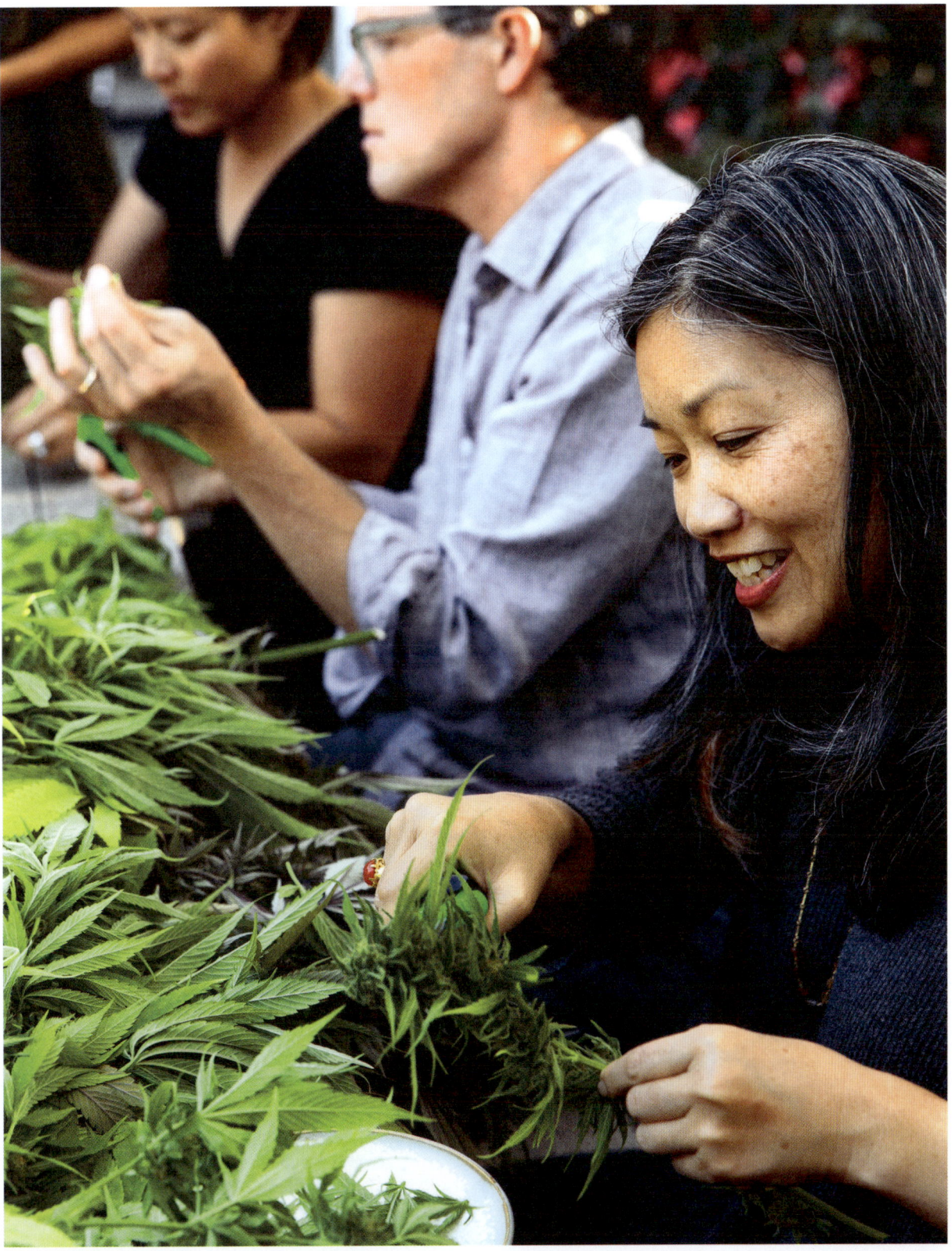

The Power of Cannabis

There are myriad health reasons to grow and consume cannabis. Remembering that the endocannabinoid system is considered the master regulatory system in the body, creating homeostasis in all the other bodily systems, there are likely health impacts for a large number of health concerns. I recommend *Cannabis Pharmacy* and *Cannabis & CBD for Health & Wellness* as two good books to help you explore your particular health condition and how cannabis can benefit you. There are excellent resources online as well. "Nurse Susan" is a free app that is simple to use. Nurse Susan is a registered cannabis nurse who offers sound advice on how to choose helpful cannabis varieties.

hybrids are constantly being introduced, as breeders refine and concentrate their genetics. Most of the cultivars found today in dispensaries, or in the illicit market, are going to be THC-dominant. The medical cannabis community has historically had more interest a balanced THC:CBD cannabinoid profile. Don't get too invested in finding the perfect cultivar. If you focus on the general type of cannabis in terms of cannabinoids and terpenes, you're going to be close to getting what you need. How you respond is perhaps the most important information of all in selecting a great type of cannabis to grow. The table on pages 20–21 outlines several common health concerns with suggestions for cannabinoids and terpenes to treat those concerns, along with some cultivar suggestions.

KNOWING WHICH PLANT IS RIGHT FOR YOU

Until recently, cannabis users used the terms *sativa* and *indica* to describe the particular effects one could expect from these respective types of cannabis. Although *sativa* is the species name of the genus *Cannabis*, it is widely accepted that there are three subspecies: *sativa sativa, sativa indica*, and *sativa ruderalis*—the subspecies important for breeders of auto-flowering cultivars only. (Auto-flowers are an emerging hybrid-type cannabis that does well in short growing seasons.) The story was that sativa-dominant weed—meaning those tall, thin-leaved, late-maturing plants that look like cannabis plants from tropical areas with their hot summers and long growing seasons—produced a heady high, a creative inclination, or an energizing experience. Conversely, indica-dominant cannabis is from the areas of central Asia and eastern Europe with their cooler summers and shorter growing seasons. Indica-leaning hybrids are said to give a relaxed high, with a sense of peaceful euphoria. Some people persist in using these terms to describe composed cannabis products for sale in dispensaries, even when these products have nothing to do with a particular cultivar's botanical origins. Sativa became an adjective for energetic highs, and indica became a shorthand for relaxing highs.

Recently, especially with the use of scientific analysis of each plant's cannabinoid and terpene profile, these terms have fallen out of fashion as surprising new information has come to light. As states have legalized cannabis, they have also mandated testing for potency and safety. The tests mandated by most states require analysis of all cannabinoids and terpenes present, total THC, and total CBD in a sample. This information has dramatically changed the expectations of growers and users alike. It turns out that the effect that can be expected from any particular cultivar is much more closely related to the cannabinoid and terpene profile than the appearance or geographical origin of the plant. So even if two

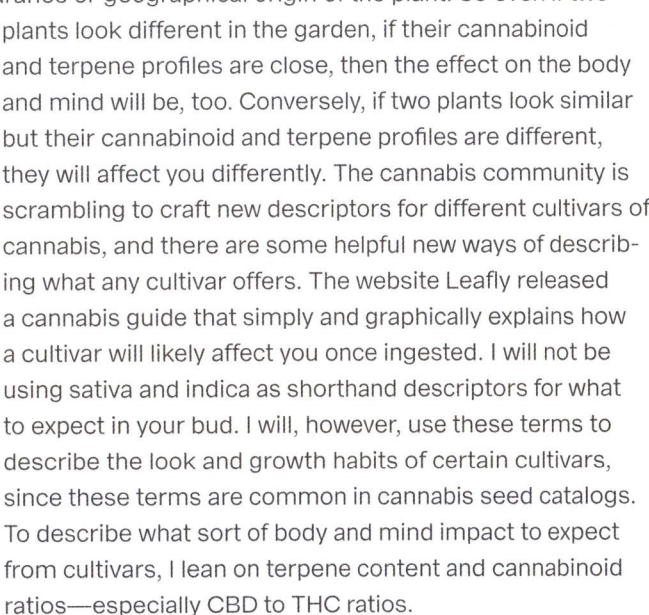
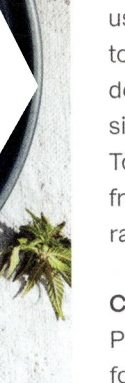

plants look different in the garden, if their cannabinoid and terpene profiles are close, then the effect on the body and mind will be, too. Conversely, if two plants look similar but their cannabinoid and terpene profiles are different, they will affect you differently. The cannabis community is scrambling to craft new descriptors for different cultivars of cannabis, and there are some helpful new ways of describing what any cultivar offers. The website Leafly released a cannabis guide that simply and graphically explains how a cultivar will likely affect you once ingested. I will not be using sativa and indica as shorthand descriptors for what to expect in your bud. I will, however, use these terms to describe the look and growth habits of certain cultivars, since these terms are common in cannabis seed catalogs. To describe what sort of body and mind impact to expect from cultivars, I lean on terpene content and cannabinoid ratios—especially CBD to THC ratios.

Cannabis vs Hemp
People have for millennia grown certain types of cannabis for particular uses: when grown for fiber and seed, it is called hemp; when grown for medicinal, mood, or spiritual uses, it is known as cannabis. Current growers are

Common Health Concerns and Treatments

HEALTH CONCERN	CANNABINOIDS	TERPENES (+ SCENT PROFILE)
Sleep	THC, CBN, CBD	Myrcene (spice/mango), Linalool (floral/warm/lavender), Caryophyllene (spice/woody/black pepper)
Pain	1:1 THC to CBD	Myrcene (spice/mango), Pinene (resinous/pine), Geraniol (floral/rose), Linalool (floral/warm/lavender)
Inflammation	THCa, CBDa, CBG, CBD, THC	Caryophyllene (spice/woody/black pepper), Myrcene (spice/mango), Linalool (floral/warm/lavender), Caryophyllene (spice/woody/black pepper)
Anxiety	CBD, CBC, CBG	Linalool (floral/warm/lavender), Myrcene (spice/mango), Caryophyllene (spice/woody/black pepper)
Euphoria/High	THC	Caryophyllene (spice/woody/black pepper), Geraniol (floral/rose), Humulene (woody/earthy/hops), Limonene (bright/lemon), Linalool (floral/warm/lavender), Myrcene (spice/mango), Pinene (resinous/pine)

CULTIVAR SUGGESTIONS	NOTES
Purple Urkle, Granddaddy Purple, Tahoe OG Kush, Purple Kush, God's Gift, Northern Lights, Ogre, 9 Pound Hammer, Remedy	For many, sleep is a big motivator for consuming cannabis. Choose a cultivar that is rich in THC and smells "purple" or woody and fruity. If you are very sensitive to THC or tend to react to THC with feelings of anxiety, look for a high-CBD variety with the terpene profile listed at left. Remedy is a good CBD cultivar with soporific terpenes. Old CBN-rich bud may be a helpful sleep aid.
Pennywise 1:1, Harlequin, Sweet Annie 1:1, Cannatonic, Dancehall, Argyle, Sweet and Sour Widow	The gold standard for treating pain is a balanced THC:CBD profile. This is the ratio that natural landrace cannabis provides. During prohibition, breeders upped the THC expression while ignoring CBD. Luckily, many breeders are now offering cultivars with a balanced THC:CBD expression. For nerve pain, look for more THC. For inflammatory pain, look for more CBD.
High THC: choose from hundreds of cultivars. **High CBD:** The Wife, Willy G's Lebanese, ACDC, Medihaze, CBD Critical Mass, Cannatonic, Royal Highness, Pennywise, CBD Blue Shark. **High CBG:** Magic Jordan, Destroyer	For inflammation, consider growing a THC-leaning cultivar and consume it raw to retain the THCa. Also helpful for inflammation is any CBD-heavy variety. CBG-rich cultivars: Magic Jordan, Panakeia, White CBG
Cannatonic, Canna-Tsu, Remedy	Especially for those who are sensitive to THC, CBD can be a best friend. A small amount of THC can be a helpful part of treating anxiety for some. Look for a cultivar with all CBD or one with several times more CBD than THC.
Blue Dream, Sour Diesel, Tangie, Melon Magic, Shangri-La are just a few of the thousands of euphoria-inducing types you can grow.	The sky is the limit in experimenting with cannabis to get high. In general, stick with cultivars that have high levels of THC relative to CBD. Terpenes will make a big difference in how you're likely to feel, so let your nose lead the way. In general, limonene and pinene offer energizing, focusing effects, while linalool and myrcene offer a sedating impact. My personal favorite is Blue Dream: I feel happy and dreamy while fully awake with this one, and it grows like magic in my garden.

intentionally cross-breeding hemp varieties with cannabis drug varieties to create all sorts of unique cultivars. It used to be that well-grown landrace cannabis (stable, natural-growing cannabis) had a pretty consistent 10 percent expression of both CBD and THC. During prohibition, the illegal weed growers selected plants that got folks really high—exhibiting THC expression of more than 30 percent with no CBD. Meanwhile, hemp grown for fiber continued to express lower overall levels of cannabinoids, with almost no THC.

Lucky for us, home growers and maverick illicit market growers have quietly been keeping unique, valuable cultivars of cannabis alive and growing. We should all be grateful for these brave souls, since many of them faced harsh punishments when their grows were discovered during prohibition. Current legal growers are building on this cultural legacy by pulling cannabis genetics from both local and global sources. Every year new varieties of cannabis are released, each with unique characteristics. And with the influx of money from the legal marketplace, huge PR budgets are in play to garner the consumer's attention and money.

There are many cultivars of cannabis available, each type offering us something unique. Consistency in the final product is important for commercial weed growers, since their livelihoods depend on giving their customers a predictable experience. But we home cannabis growers have more flexibility and can take a risk on a new cannabis plant without breaking our budgets. We get to be explorers in our own gardens!

Where You Live Matters

Cannabis sativa grows in just about any climate that humans have traditionally inhabited. Cannabis is found on every continent except Antarctica, and it will grow in every state in the United States. From Hawaii to Alaska, Maine to Arizona—there is a cannabis cultivar that will grow where you live. As long you provide rich soil, lots of sun, and enough water, there is very likely going to be a cultivar that you can grow outside. That said, it is important to consider the specific climate zone you'll be growing in to choose the best weed to plant in your outdoor growing space. I address the specific needs of your cannabis plants to grow well outside in chapters 3 and 4. In this chapter, our aim is to zoom out a bit and understand what our place on the globe is and how this narrows our choices of cannabis plants.

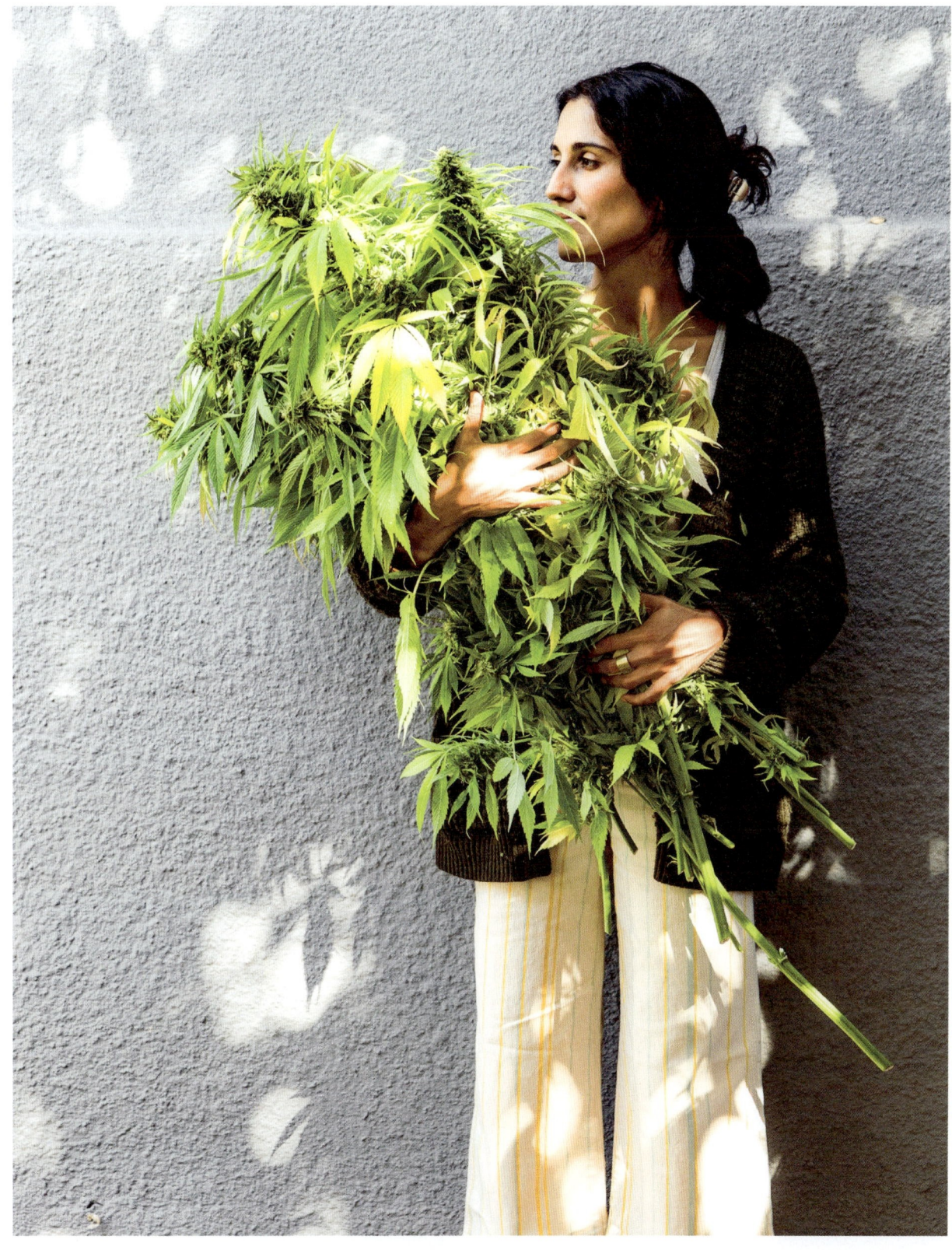

What's My USDA or Sunset Garden Zone?

Start with the climate zone you are in. There are three climate zone systems that are helpful to determine the climate you live and grow in: the global Köppen Climate Classification, the USDA climate zone and, for some of us, the Sunset Western Garden Climate Zones. I live and garden in the cool summer, mild winter climate of the Bay Area in California. As such, in the Köppen Climate Classification system, this is Csb, or Mediterranean climate. According to the USDA, I'm in Zone 10a. But since I garden in California with its huge number of microclimates, the USDA zones are not very useful. I rely mostly on the Sunset Western Garden Climate Zones, and my garden falls in zone 17 for this guide. The Sunset zones are available for the western half of the United States. For those of you living east of the Rockies, the USDA zones are helpful enough, especially when combined with information from the Köppen Climate Classification system.

Local Climate Challenges

Below are some common climate challenges you may face in your area and the cannabis plants that will work best for you. Weed cultivars come and go, so I focus instead on what growth characteristics to look for in a plant. I recommend sourcing seeds from local companies

CLIMATE CHALLENGES	PLANT ISSUES	BEST PLANT CHOICES
Cool, moist fall	Powdery mildew, bud rot	Mold-resistant indica-dominant, fast-maturing cultivars
Hot, dry summer	Mites, drought	Sativa-dominant, late-maturing bud
Hot, humid summer	Powdery mildew	Mold-resistant sativa-dominant
Small seasonal fluctuations	Lanky growth, small bud	Sativa-dominant, auto-flowering
Short summer	Immature bud at first frost	Auto-flowering, fast-maturing cultivars

if possible, because they know the targeted needs of their region's growers. Make some new friends in your local cannabis-growing community to get more specific cultivar recommendations.

CHOOSING WHERE TO PLANT

The next question to consider is where in your garden you will be growing your cannabis plants. Will you be growing in a container, in a raised bed, or in the ground? (For more on the differences among these three choices, see page 34.) This is helpful information to know before selecting a seed or clone, the two choices of cannabis plant starts (see page 66). In general, cannabis plants grown from seed (seedlings) are larger and more vigorous than cannabis grown from clones. If you have rich, well-worked garden soil, then a seedling is the best choice for maximum vigor and harvest. Another plus of growing from seed is that there are lots of varieties from which to choose, they are easily purchased online, and they carry less risk of disease transfer than clones. If you will be growing in a container, then a clone may offer the best balance of good growth and convenience. Raised beds will accommodate either seedlings or clones. Gardeners who don't want to deal with starting seeds will be best served by planting a clone.

DETERMINING HOW MANY PLANTS TO GROW

The last factor to consider when choosing the best cannabis for your garden is to decide how many plants to grow. First, establish two key things: (1) what is legally allowed in your area and (2) how much space do you have?

What Are the Laws in Your State?

Let's consider the legality issue first. Before you grow cannabis in your garden, it's important to find out whether or not it's legal. Cannabis can grow in nearly every part of the world, and each country has a different set of laws that govern the possession and growing of this plant. Uruguay and Canada have both completely legalized cannabis. Several other nations— New Zealand being one of them—are poised to consider legalization in the near future. However, in the United States, this gentle herb is still federally illegal and classified as a schedule 1 drug. But 99 percent of US cannabis arrests are made under state law, so it's important to know what your state and local laws are in addition to your country's federal laws. Some states have legalized recreational cannabis cultivation, and some haven't. And to make it even more confusing, even in states where it is legal to grow cannabis—such as California—there are certain restrictions that override this general statewide legality. For example, if I were to bring some of my garden-grown cannabis to a national park, a post office, a school, onto a

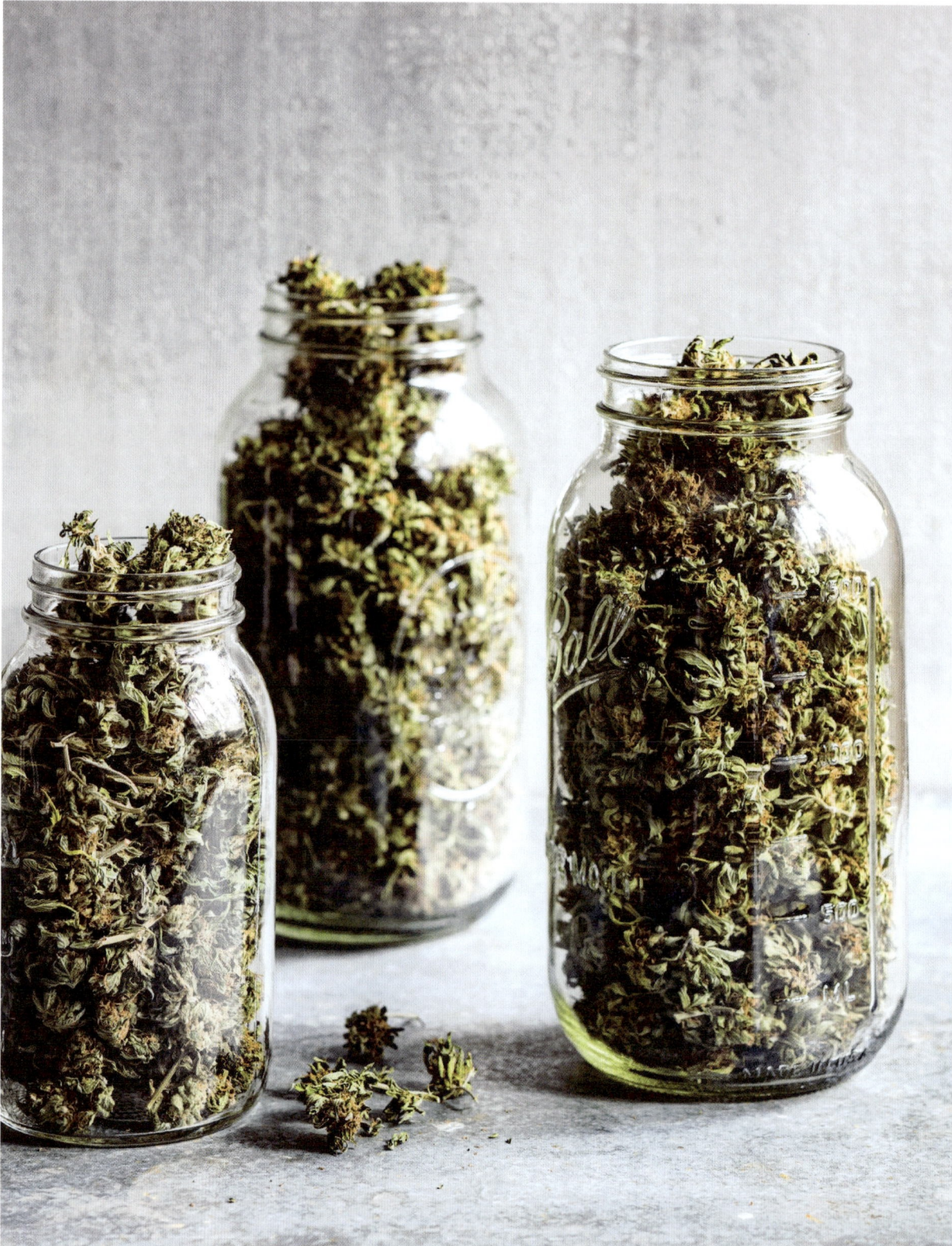

In my garden . . .

This past season I grew five plants total—two in 20-gallon grow pots and three in the ground. My hope was to get a wide variety of health effects from my grow. I grew two Abacus plants because I wanted a CBD-only variety—plus, someone had given me seeds. I grew Pennywise 1:1 because it is a balanced CBD:THC variety and smells bright like a sea breeze, with lemon and pine scents. Pennywise 1:1 is fabulous at reducing my pain and helps ward off impending migraines—it's become my go-to bud. I grew Blue Dream because it is a high THC-yielding plant and a great grower in my area—plus I love how it makes me feel. It was a great season, yielding a whopping 4½ pounds of dry bud.

boat, or to an airport, it's a potential legal problem. Why? Because these are federal lands, even if they are located within the state of California. Under Proposition 64, also known as the Adult Use of Marijuana Act, California cities can ban the home cannabis grows even if they are legally allowed by the state.

There are commonsense age requirements in play in most states. For example, in California you have to be twenty-one or older to grow cannabis at home. If an underage person grows even one cannabis plant, this can have big consequences. I encourage you to do a little research and get to know the state and local laws where you live and garden. A good source for up-to-date information is NORML—the National Organization for the Reform of Marijuana Laws—a well-respected nonprofit cannabis legalization advocacy organization. Their website has a state-by-state map with up-to-the-minute information on the legality and growing of cannabis. There are international chapters of NORML as well, for those readers living in countries around our beautiful globe. For those of you who are cannabis-loving people living in a culture or country different from the one in which you were raised, be mindful of the local social norms and laws regarding cannabis cultivation and use.

How Much Space Will You Need?

Another factor in deciding how many plants to grow is how much space you have outside. Whether you grow in a pot, in a raised bed, or in the ground, cannabis needs ample room to grow and at least six hours of full sun per day. A typical cannabis plant will reach 6 to 9-plus feet tall and nearly as wide at maturity, depending on growing conditions, and needs a nice big area of soil to reach its best potential. Look at all of your available spaces—a sunny deck, an area of lawn that you can dig up and enrich, a raised vegetable bed, even a chunk of concrete or patio; any one of these areas could be an excellent place to grow cannabis. A way to get a quick read on whether or not you'll have enough space for cannabis plants is to walk out into your garden. Stand right where you think a cannabis plant would grow well, then put out your arms, turn around in a circle, and look up. Do you see sky? Great. Did your hands move in a circle freely with no obstructions? Also great. This will be a good spot to grow one cannabis plant—because a mature cannabis plant at harvest will be about the size of an adult human. Repeat this exercise for each spot you think would work.

How Much to Grow

Finally, a word about yield. The harvest per healthy cannabis plant grown outside in the sun is up to 1 pound of dried, cured bud. This amount can vary considerably, but this is an achievable, though high, benchmark for what to expect. If you're used to thinking about cannabis in terms of grams, this is about 450 grams of dried bud. That's a lot of weed! For perspective, a typical joint weighs about half a gram. So, as you decide how many plants to grow, consider how much weed you'd like to harvest as a key piece of information.

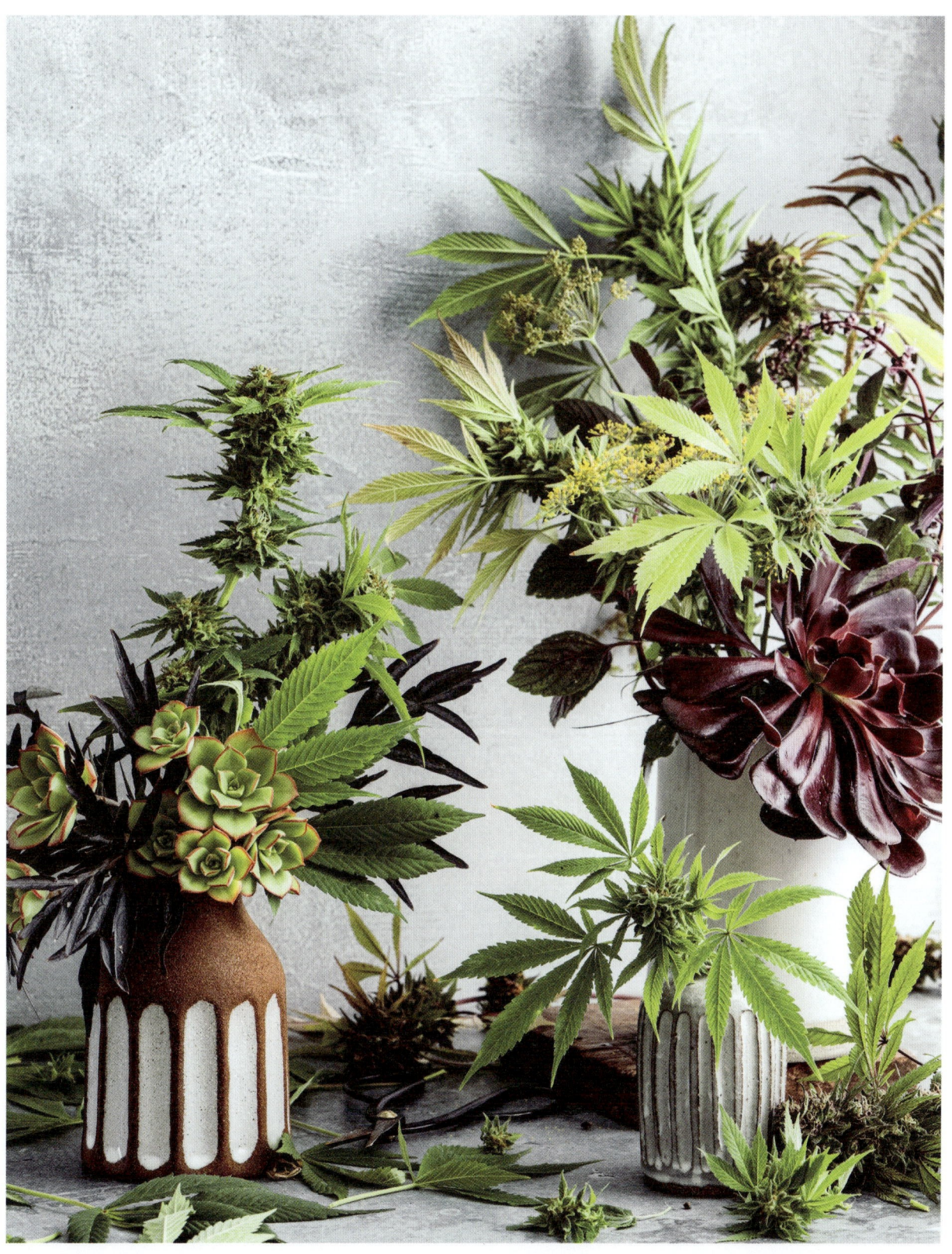

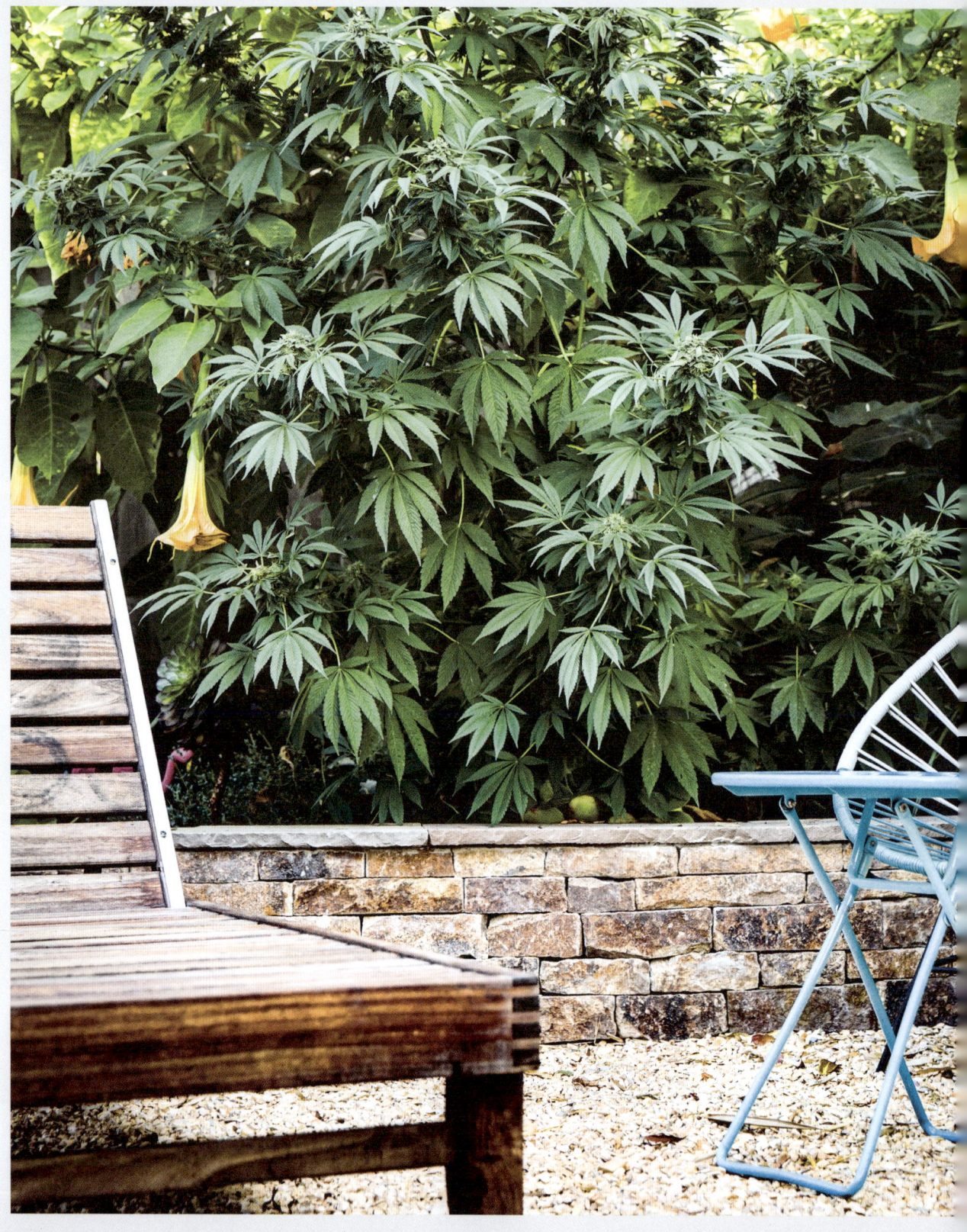

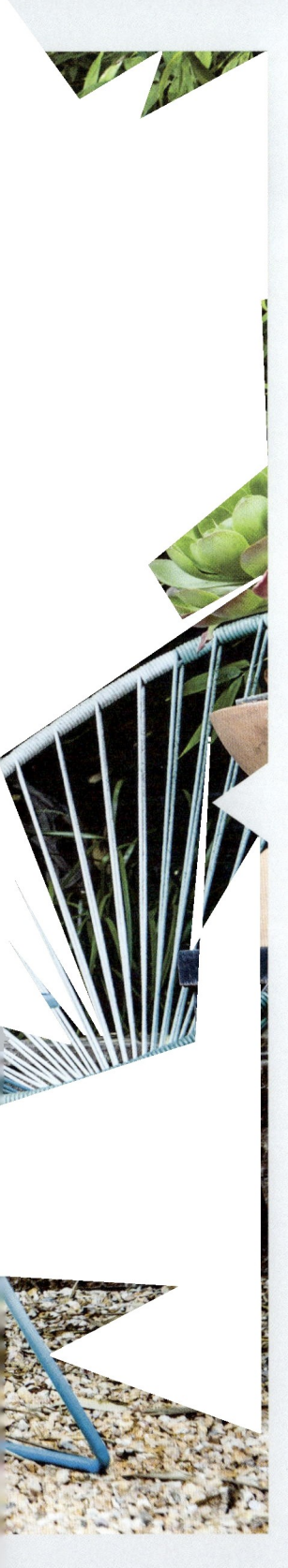

CHAPTER 2

Designing Your Garden Space with Cannabis

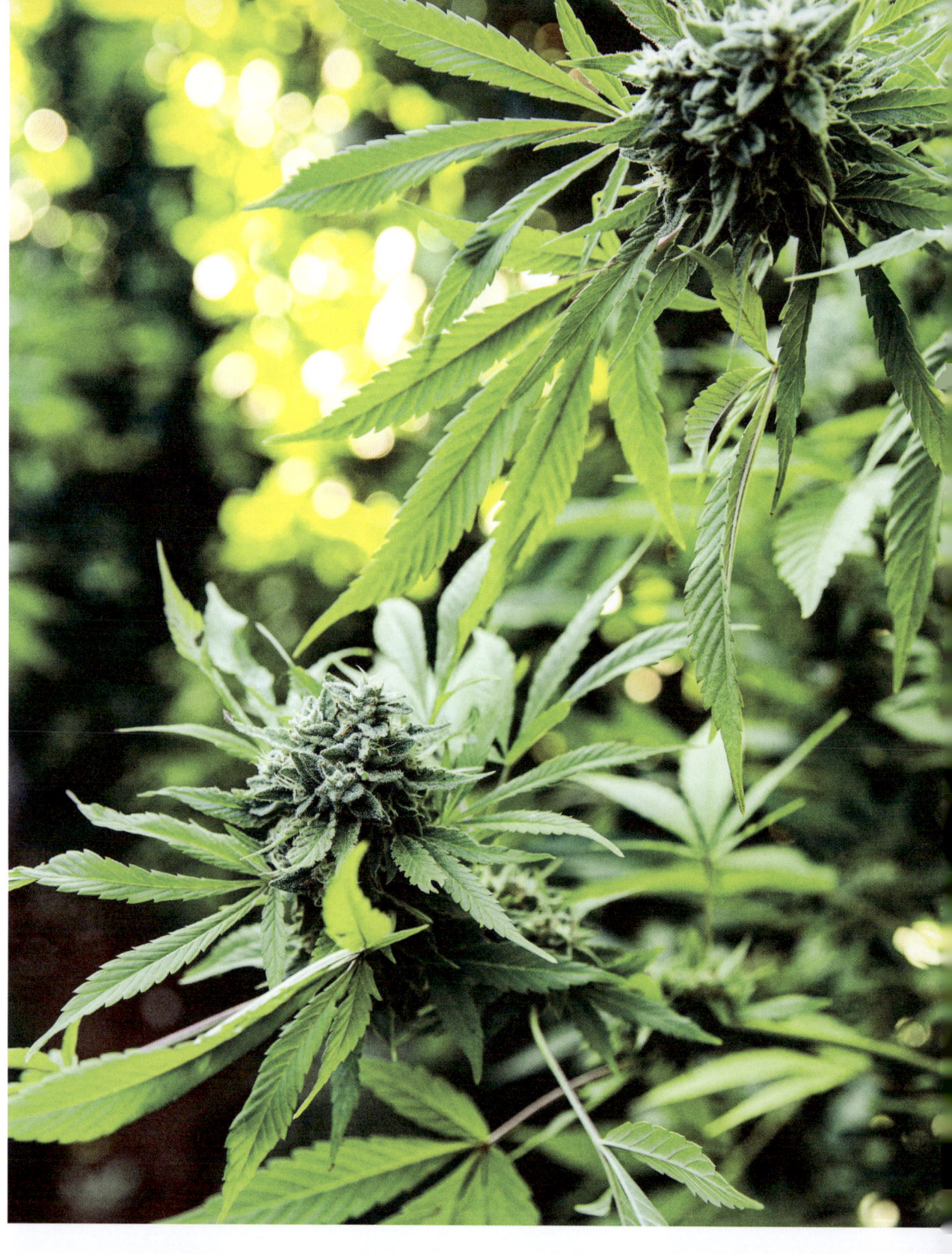

When you act in your space—however small or big—to craft a healthy environment for your plants, you are a gardener. When you think ahead through the coming seasons and imagine the plants you can grow, you are thinking like a gardener. Whether you have a vast estate, a backyard bed, or a tiny porch, growing a plant with care makes you a gardener. One container filled with soil, planted, watered, and nurtured through its seasons is a garden. The word "garden" has its origin in the Latin *hortus gardinus*, which describes a place of enclosure for growing useful and beautiful plants. Gardens are where the human creative spirit works to craft a natural space into a new thing, a place with purpose and productivity in mind. The best gardeners work with nature, not against it. When we work with the gifts of our natural surroundings rather than fighting them, we are better gardeners. I advocate organic gardening practices, leaning heavily on good design, proper site selection, and optimal soil health.

One of the most creative aspects of gardening is to design the garden space to your liking. When you design your garden space, you become—at least a little—a garden designer. There are many styles from which to gather inspiration. Each culture around the world has its own ways of gardening, stemming from the climate and sociological context in which it arose. Some of the most famous gardens throughout time are the walled gardens of Persia, the peaceful Zen gardens of Japan, the classical gardens of China, charming English cottage gardens, and the stately formal gardens of Europe. There are large numbers of publications and degree programs devoted to garden design. However, this chapter offers one central encouragement: cannabis works in just about any sunny garden space. No matter what your garden's current style (or lack thereof), you can add cannabis. And perhaps you can use cannabis as an incentive to improve the overall look and feel of your garden. Looking ahead to a healthy harvest is a great way to gain motivation to make your garden a productive, beautiful space for you and your plants. Trust me—when your friends hear you talk about your huge green weed plant, they will want to stop by for a visit. That's a great incentive to get your garden designer game on.

Take a moment to see your garden space with the mindset of a garden designer, and you will be rewarded by its usefulness and appeal in the future. One way to step into the role of garden designer is to correlate it to an activity you've likely had some experience with—arranging the look and feel of a room in your home. In fact, garden designers often use concepts and language borrowed from architecture and interior design to do their work. They think of gardens as having walls, floors, beds, focal points, ceilings—but instead of manufactured building materials, they use plants, soil, lumber, and stone. Like interior designers, you can coordinate the look of your garden rooms by grouping plants by color, size, and texture—but instead of fabrics, furniture, and paint, you can use flowers, fruit, leaves, and branches for your work. Gardeners think like parents, imagining the whole life cycle of the plants they grow, from seed to flower. Gardeners have the unique, added constraint of working with living things—plants. Personally, I love this aspect of gardening the most. We aren't in control—we influence, we nurture. What a great life lesson: there is nothing perfect in gardening, but there is enormous abundance and surprise.

THREE COMMON GARDEN DESIGNS

Let's use three common garden types to gain confidence and inspiration: the container garden, the raised bed garden, and the garden room. Each of these three types of gardens will adapt to your individual style, whether it is a kitchen garden, wabi-sabi, cottage garden, minimalist and modern, lush and tropical, formal and ordered, or meandering and wild.

Cannabis in a Container

Constraint can be a catalyst for creativity. Perhaps the only spot you have for gardening is on a deck or patio. That's no problem—let it be a motivation rather than a limitation. Allow the restriction of your limited space to become a catalyst for your creativity by gardening in containers. You can grow healthy, full-size cannabis in a container. The container garden is the

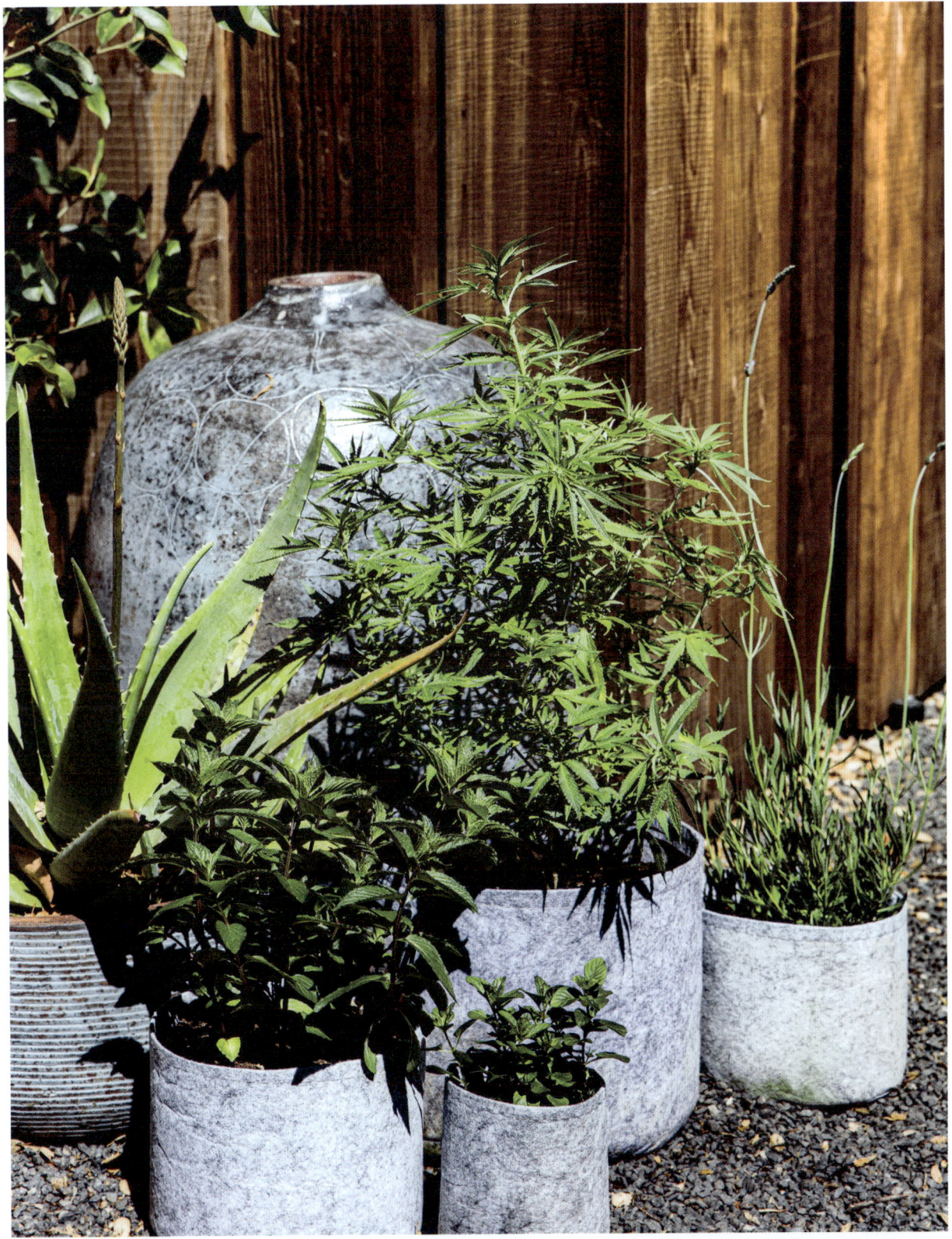

simplest garden of all and is an ideal place for the beginning cannabis grower. It is also a high art form, perhaps most elegantly expressed in bonsai gardens—each little container holding a garden scene in perfectly scaled miniature. You can grow full-size, high-quality cannabis on a sunny deck off your apartment or on a concrete patio in your backyard. If you have access to a rooftop, this can be an excellent spot for cannabis container gardening because of its full-sun conditions. Even for those of you who have larger garden plots, a container garden may be the right choice. The single most important consideration for placing your container is ample sunlight. A plus for growing weed in a container is that you can move the cannabis plant to the light, adjusting placement as the seasons change to maximize your plant's sun exposure. This may be a great solution for those of you with shady yards but sunny spots on a deck. Cannabis needs at least six or more hours of direct sunlight per day to grow well—and more is better. Of course, this is only when cannabis is actually growing, so if you have a spot that receives less than this amount in late fall through spring, that's not an issue. If you have very lightly dappled shade and the plant will receive eight or more hours of this exposure per day, this will work, too.

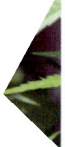

Once you've chosen a sunny spot, consider what type and size container to use. Cannabis is a large, fast-growing annual. Its roots are vigorous and will fill a large volume of soil, so a big container will allow for a full-size cannabis plant. *Using fresh, high-quality planting mix is key to growing healthy cannabis in a container, no matter what size planter you choose.* Every penny invested in good planting mix is money well spent. Containers are usually sold in standard sizes and are measured in units of volume, such as gallons or liters. The minimum size for any container should be 5 gallons. I grew plants in 15-gallon pots this past season and had full-size plants—both were more than 7 feet tall at harvest. Commercial growers will sometimes have 100-gallon grow bags for enormous cannabis plants. Good drainage is another very important consideration. Be sure to inspect the bottoms of the pots you want to use to ensure there are drainage holes.

If you have room for a few planters, consider creating an attractive grouping. The rule of three is a good design tip to create an appealing cluster of containers.

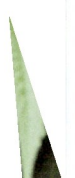

Try planting some mint, lemon verbena, or lavender (see page 47) in planters of the same material as your cannabis plant for the ultimate cannabis tisane—or herbal tea—planter garden. For a more cohesive look, purchase or make planters of the same material, allowing the beauty of the plants to create visual interest. Put these smaller planters on the sunward side of your cannabis plant's larger container, so every plant receives the sun that they need to grow well. Grouping containers together will help keep the soil cooler, especially in those containers that are shaded by the pots in front.

There are several different types of containers from which to choose to house your cannabis plant. Let's explore the characteristics of the more commonly available containers, considering the pros and cons of each.

Terra-cotta. These red-hued earthenware planters are a classic choice for containers. There is good reason for this. Terra-cotta means "baked earth" in Italian and is an apt description of what this material is. The low-fire clay used in this type of pot creates excellent conditions for your cannabis plant's roots, since the walls of this natural earthenware material are porous and allow the soil to breathe and remain cool. Unglazed terra-cotta pots have a warm red-orange color; glazed terra-cotta comes in a rainbow of colors. While simple pots are inexpensive, the larger or more specially glazed pots can be costly.

> **Pros:** Terra-cotta planters provide excellent conditions for soil health, are readily available, come in many different shapes and colors, and offer visual appeal for most garden styles.

> **Cons:** Terra-cotta containers that are large enough for cannabis can be heavy. Because of their porous walls, terra-cotta pots are prone to cracking during harsh winter freeze/thaw cycles and need to be emptied of their soil during the off-season and stored inside for longevity. If you live in a climate with mild winters, you can safely leave your terra-cotta pots outside with no fear of freeze/thaw damage.

Felt planter. Commercial cannabis growers have used felt planters for a while, especially for covert outdoor cannabis grow operations. These felt bags are called grow bags in the cannabis trade, and home gardeners have adopted this term widely as well. These containers are usually made from felted recycled plastic but may be made from felted natural fibers that have been molded or stitched to form a pot. No drainage holes are needed for these bags, since they are naturally wicking and porous.

Pros: Inexpensive, lightweight, and with excellent porosity, felt planters make a great choice for cannabis container growing. Because felt breathes so well, the soil ball remains cool, and there is no hard surface for the roots to contact—so no root-bound plants. Look for handles on these planters if you plan to move them once planted.

Cons: Felt planters can discolor from soil and water leaching into the material. Bags made from natural fibers may have lower durability, because constant contact with wet soil promotes decay, but they are all-natural and compostable. Plants grown in felt planters will require more frequent watering, since the fabric is porous and water will evaporate more quickly.

Ceramic. Made from a high-temperature–fired clay, ceramic pots are nearly always finished with a glaze and come in a large array of decorative finishes. They are strong but thinner-walled than terra-cotta. Look for pots with drainage holes.

Pros: There are beautiful ceramic planters available for those interested in a particular look for their pots. Ceramic pots are moisture retentive, since the planter walls are less permeable to the air than are those of unglazed terra-cotta. Ceramic pots provide good conditions for soil overall.

Cons: Ceramic pots that are large enough to host a full season of cannabis growing will be heavy and can be expensive. Cannabis roots may begin to circle as they hit the inner edge of the ceramic pot and look for more soil, potentially creating less than perfect conditions toward the end of the grow season. Dark glazes may create high-temperature conditions for the root-ball, especially in hot, sunny climates. Although ceramic pots are more weather resistant than most unglazed terra-cotta, they will need to be emptied and stored inside in harsh winter climates to preserve their life span.

Plastic. These pots can be made of any type of plastic or fiberglass, may be single- or double-walled, and are available in many colors, sizes, and shapes.

Pros: Plastic is inexpensive and readily available. These pots are moisture retentive, since their walls are impermeable to water and air. Plastic pots are durable and can be left outside during winter without fear of cracking, although they will have a longer life span if they are protected from harsh winters.

Cons: Plastic made from petrochemicals is non-renewable and non-compostable, so plastic pots are a poor choice for environmental sustainability. Plastic made from renewable sources is a better choice. Plastic and fiberglass pots are moisture-proof, so roots may circle the insides of the pots as they reach maturity.

Metal. Metal pots are usually made from aluminum or steel.

Pros: Metals pots are lightweight relative to terra-cotta or ceramic and are very durable. Like any nonporous material, they are moisture retentive.

Cons: Metal conducts heat, so this type of pot may provide high swings of heat to the roots of your cannabis plant. Steel containers are usually on the expensive side. Metal pots are moisture-proof, so roots may circle the insides of the pots as they reach maturity.

Wood. Wooden containers are manufactured with various types of wood, often from bamboo or old wine barrels that have been cut in half. If you plan to use a wooden planter, make sure it has adequate drainage holes.

Pros: A wooden planter provides good conditions for soil, since it offers permeability to air and moisture. Wooden pots are relatively durable, especially if they are made from rot-resistant cedar or redwood.

Cons: Wooden planters can be costly, especially finely crafted planters or ones that use more expensive woods. Be sure to avoid pots made with chemically treated wood, since cannabis can absorb these chemicals into its cell structure.

Concrete. These planters are made from Portland cement and an aggregate. The aggregate can be mineral or natural fiber—even hemp is used to make concrete (hempcrete).

Pros: Concrete planters are great if you're looking for a modern, minimalist design. They are durable and strong and will last for many growing seasons.

Cons: Concrete is heavy and usually expensive relative to other planters. Brand-new concrete planters may leach alkali into the soil, causing the soil pH to rise; this can weaken your cannabis plant.

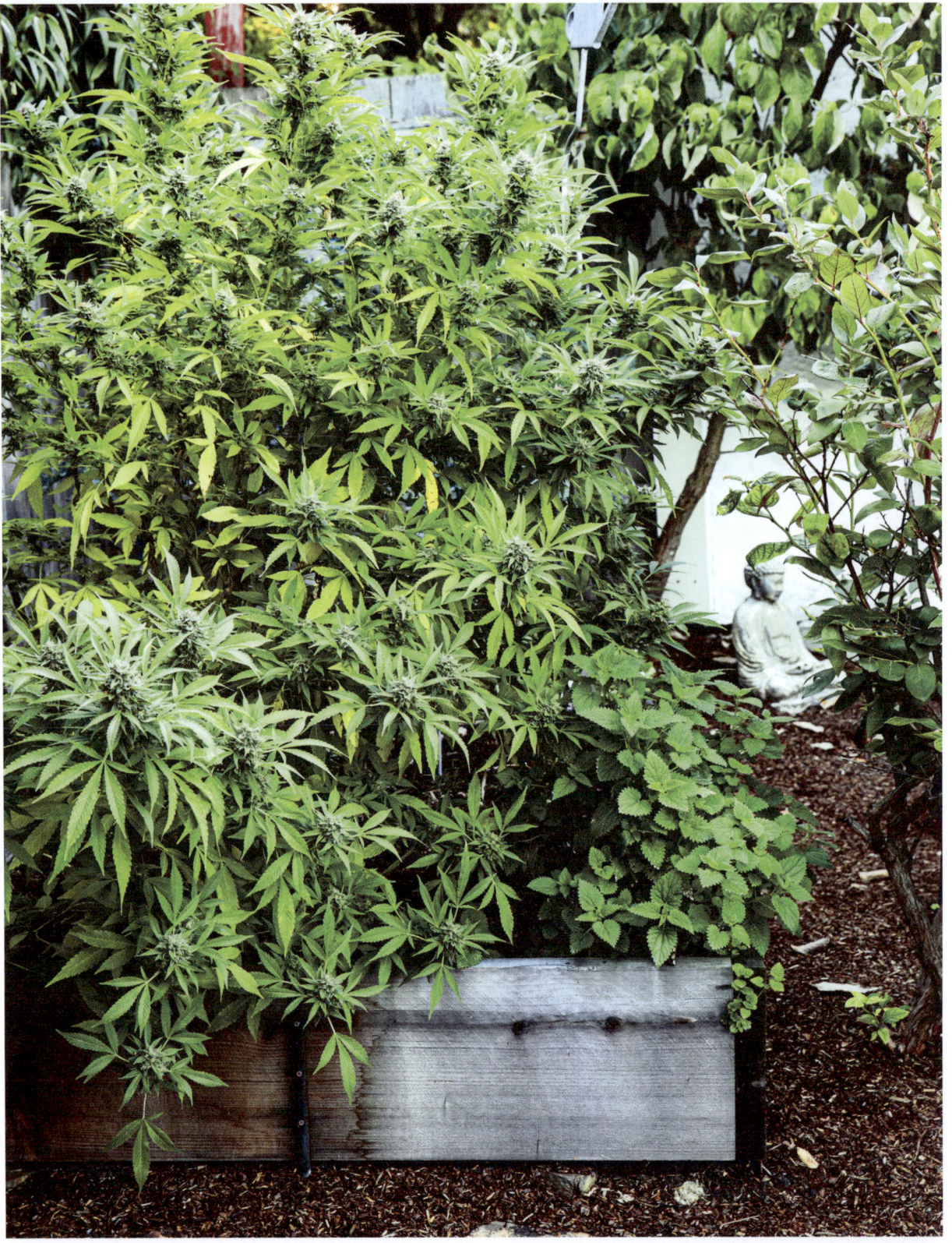

Other materials. Hypertufa, fiberglass, raffia, cane, glass, cardboard, woven fabrics—basically anything nontoxic and water resistant that you use to keep soil in place for the growing season—can become a planter for your cannabis.

Cannabis in a Raised Bed

If you have a bit of land, even a small backyard plot, you can expand your cannabis growing space to include raised beds. What is a raised bed? The concept of a raised bed will likely be familiar to anyone who grows vegetables. It is a wide, open-bottomed structure, used to create a space above the ground level and is filled with rich soil mix. Raised beds are often used for growing annual vegetables—although any plant can grow in a raised bed. Raised beds are usually constructed of rot-resistant wood or metal but can be made from stone, concrete, brick, caged rocks, or other durable materials. Since cannabis is an annual crop, it makes sense to grow it in an area where you might also grow a healthy tomato plant—both require similar conditions. Raised beds are excellent options for steep ground, too, since they can be built to act as terraces on slopes. They are also wonderful for drought-prone areas, because they offer a focused area to water plants. And for gardening in very wet climates, raised beds offer superb drainage, which cannabis needs. One other benefit of raised beds for cool, wet winter climates (think Seattle and British Columbia) is that the soil in a raised bed will warm quickly in the spring, allowing for the best soil conditions for planting cannabis. I love raised beds for the flexibility they offer in creating ideal soil conditions.

In my garden . . .

Where I live and grow, our soils are clay type. Over the years, I've continually amended my garden's soil, and the overall fertility and structure is much improved with annual additions of compost. But when I want fresh, deep, rich soil for my nutrient-hungry annual crops, I love my raised bed. I have learned that many fast-growing plants do best when planted in fresh soil, and cannabis is one of them.

As with any planting scheme for your cannabis, be sure that your cannabis will have full sun and freedom from encroaching tree roots. As you imagine where to best situate your cannabis plants, use your own body (see page 28) to help visualize the size of your plant at maturity. Then consider the impact it will have on the surrounding plants in the same raised bed.

If you have a new raised bed filled with rich, fresh planting mix, then you are ready to plant your cannabis directly into the soil at planting time in your area. If you have an existing raised bed in which you've grown plants during previous seasons, you will need to amend or replace some of the existing planting mix. (See chapter 3 to learn more about the soil requirements for cannabis growing.)

Cannabis is a fast-growing plant, each requiring up to 16 square feet of space at maturity—think 4 by 4 feet, with 2 feet of soil depth. For all growers outside of the tropics, we need to be mindful of the shadows cast by plants onto their botanical neighbors. For those growing in the Northern Hemisphere, position taller plants northward of shorter plants; reverse this in the Southern Hemisphere.

When you first place your new plant in the soil, though, it will be small and will look a little isolated in the raised bed. I suggest that you plant a quick-maturing companion crop to take advantage of the space that your cannabis will eventually grow into. Try growing a crop of lettuce, arugula, radishes, or quick-maturing cooking greens in the area around the baby cannabis plant. By the time your cannabis plant is large enough to crowd out these annuals, you will already have harvested them—a gardening twofer. Known as biointensive gardening, this is a familiar concept to many and is often referred to as French intensive gardening or square foot gardening. It is a space- and resource-efficient method of gardening that translates well to the cannabis gardener's needs. The concept of intensively planted raised beds is not uniquely French and has been utilized by many gardening and farming cultures around the world.

Cannabis in a Perennial Garden

I have a lovely little cottage garden in my backyard. More accurately, my whole backyard—25 by 30 feet total—*is* a cottage garden. It's just the right size for me to treat it like a single garden room. For those of you with more land in which to garden, you may have garden areas such as a front yard, side yard, or backyard—each with its own light, soil, trees, shrubs, and hardscaping. Many gardeners have space in their landscape dedicated to perennial beds. These are areas bordering a lawn or patio

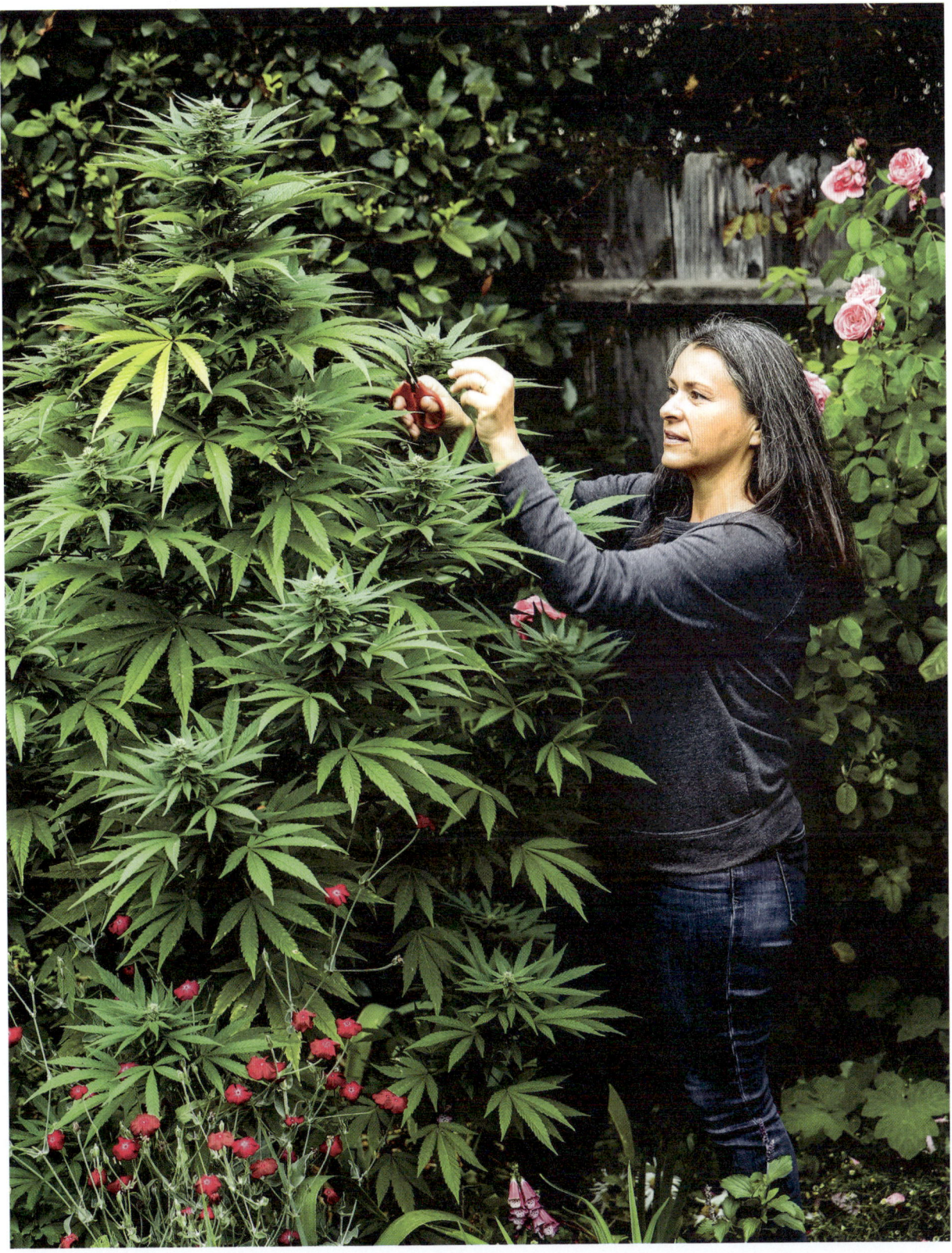

that have a variety of long-lived flowers, grasses, and shrubs. The perennial bed is often densely planted to create a seasonally changing tapestry of beauty and usefulness, especially when it contains fruiting shrubs and herbs for the kitchen.

A perennial bed with rich soil can easily welcome a couple of cannabis plants, size allowing. When planting cannabis in an existing perennial bed, there are three important considerations: space, soil quality, and sun. Sound familiar? These are the same exact considerations that we have already discussed in the container garden and raised bed sections above. I will highlight here the special issues you need to think about in an existing perennial bed. For those who garden in areas where deer are abundant, take care to protect your cannabis plants from them. Deer will happily nibble on weed babies.

The space. Look at your perennial bed and find a spot where you think a full-size cannabis plant would work. As before, walk out to the spot, put your arms out, and turn in a circle (see page 28). Will a cannabis plant grow here without being crowded out by a shrub or tree? Is there full sun exposure? At full size, will the cannabis plant shade out a plant behind it? If all of these things seem good, the next task is to examine the ground you'll be planting the cannabis in. Are there smaller plants growing within a 5-foot circle of the cannabis plant's center? If so, they will be impacted by dense shade toward the end of the summer, so be mindful of these plants' needs. Investigate the soil in which you'll be planting the cannabis. Unless you have been amending and tending your garden soil for a while or if you are lucky enough to live in an area with naturally fertile, well-draining soil, you'll need to amend the soil with compost prior to the planting season. (See chapter 3 for more specifics on composting.) Do a little digging to be sure that there aren't roots from surrounding shrubs or trees that may hinder the growth of your cannabis plant. If there are, plan on digging out these roots to create a nice, loose area of soil for your cannabis.

Companion plants. Once you've located the right spot in your perennial bed for your cannabis plant—or more than one if you have room— consider what you can plant around the cannabis plant. Think of both the look and the usefulness of companion plants for your weed. If you live in a mild winter area such as California or the South, you have the luxury of time—via the year-long gardening potential. This will enable you to plant something for winter and early spring beauty before you plant your weed.

In my garden . . .

I garden all year long in my mild-winter Bay Area backyard. I have an area in the ground for two full-size cannabis plants and have several months of growing season before I plant the cannababies in late April. This fall, I planted a couple hundred spring blooming bulbs and seeds of the California native spring ephemeral baby blue eyes (*Nemophila menziesii*). These will be bloomed out and dormant by the time my cannabis plant is tall enough to shade them. This garden has beauty and productivity throughout the year. Another option for my cannabis space is to grow sweet peas—one of my favorites. These are spring/summer bloomers in much of the temperate world, but in my garden, they are an early spring bloomer. My trick is to plant 4-inch pots of sweet pea plants in late fall. Come early spring, these well-rooted sweet peas clamber up a temporary structure and start to bloom. By the time the sweet peas have moved beyond their peak, the young cannabis plant will be ready to grow and shine. And there's a bonus: sweet peas—like all legumes—add nitrogen to the soil, providing a boost to the fast-growing cannabis plant.

Cannabis in a Cutting Garden

For those of you with cutting gardens—welcome to your new floral arrangement superstar: cannabis. A cutting garden is simply one in which flowers are grown for cutting or for use in floral arrangements to grace your home. A cutting garden is a little different from a perennial bed in that its primary purpose is to be productive, rather than beautiful. Not to say that a well-designed cutting bed can't be beautiful, but a cutting bed is often arranged with more function in mind than visual appeal alone— annuals planted in rows, with air space between plants to prioritize the long stems and floral production desired in a vase. Annual cutting gardens are ideally set up to accommodate cannabis, because cannabis shares the same cultural conditions of many popular annual cutting flowers such as cosmos, sunflowers, zinnias, cornflowers, larkspur, poppies, coreopsis, and ranunculus. As long as you remember just how large the mature cannabis plant will become and place it appropriately in the cutting garden, you'll be in great shape. Cannabis is wonderful and unexpected when used in floral arrangements. As cannabis grows, it produces many side branches that can be easily incorporated into bouquets. Weed holds up beautifully in a vase, adding structure, texture, and je ne sais quoi to your bouquet. For those of you living in an area in which outdoor cannabis growing is legally allowed but is still new, consider cultivating cannabis in the midst of similar-looking plants to ease this notorious beauty into your landscape. Some plants that offer the appropriate scale to accompany cannabis include cleomes, sunflowers, tithonia, large coreopsis, bush zinnias, gladiolas, and flowering tobacco.

Cannabis in an Herb Garden

Cannabis is perhaps best thought of as a kitchen herb, so it's a natural fit for any herb garden. It bears repeating that cannabis is large relative to most nontree garden plants. But if you allow for the majestic proportions of cannabis, it is a perfect fit for an herb garden. Cannabis is delicious in the teapot and pairs nicely with several standard garden herbs. Fresh

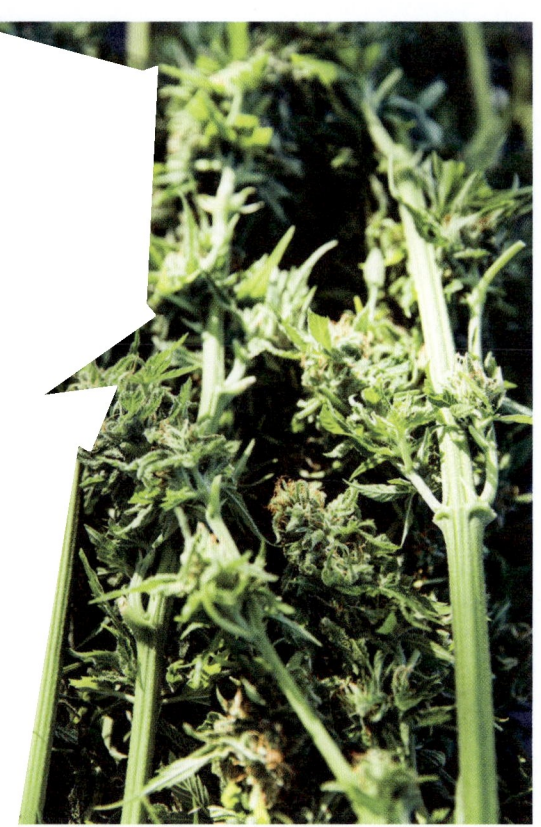

cannabis leaves make an excellent tisane (herbal tea) with soothing, calming properties. There are several easy-to-grow companion plants that you can harvest and infuse with cannabis for a delicious beverage. My favorite garden plants for this use are lemon verbena, thyme, German chamomile, and lavender. I especially love spearmint; I grow several types of mint, and all are welcome additions to the teapot along with cannabis (see page 175).

Best Herbal Companion Plants

Lemon verbena, or *Aloysia citrodora* (USDA zone 8–10), is a tall airy shrub, native to western South America, with deliciously scented, pointed leaves. It sheds its leaves in late fall in my mild-winter garden and is one of the last to leaf out in the spring. It does well with a light winter pruning to maintain plant vigor and to control size. The leaves are ready to use in tisanes as soon as they are formed and will remain useful throughout the season, until they begin to shrivel and fall off the plant at the end of the growth season. Luckily, lemon verbena leaves dry easily and can offer a delightful reminder of summer during the dark days of winter. Plant lemon verbena in a full-sun spot with room to grow slowly over the years. They do well with regular watering but are tolerant of heat and drought. They are remarkably pest resistant, due in part to the high essential oil content of their leaves and the leaves' slightly rough texture. As an upright grower, lemon verbena shrubs are perfect to underplant with low-growing herbs and flowers. This tender perennial may be grown in a container and brought inside in cold winter climates.

Mint. Cannabis and mint together make a delicious tisane. Try growing mint around your cannabis. While there are many members of the mint family, when most folks think of mint, they mean spearmint. Most mints possess an unmistakably fresh, cool scent profile. While there are hundreds of varieties of mint, they all possess similar growth habits. Mints are easy-going, low-growing (up to 3 feet tall but usually shorter) garden plants that enjoy moist soil and dappled shade to full sun. They are happiest in rich soil but are tolerant of many soil types. They have tender, green crenulated leaves that cover the spreading stolons (creeping horizontal plant stems). A word of caution is needed if you intend to plant mint in the ground: they are wanderers and will spread to seek out ideal sun and moisture. For this reason, many gardeners are wary of planting mints directly in their gardens, since mints are truly rambunctious wherever there is abundant moisture. I live in a dry summer climate and thus allow several types of mint to ramble all over my garden. I keep their growth in check with occasional removal—they are easy to rip out of the soil. One of my favorite mints for the teapot (or the cocktail shaker) is Kentucky Colonel spearmint—a classic in a mint julep. Chocolate mint is also a richly scented, delicious mint and accompanies the deep, musky flavor of cannabis with flair.

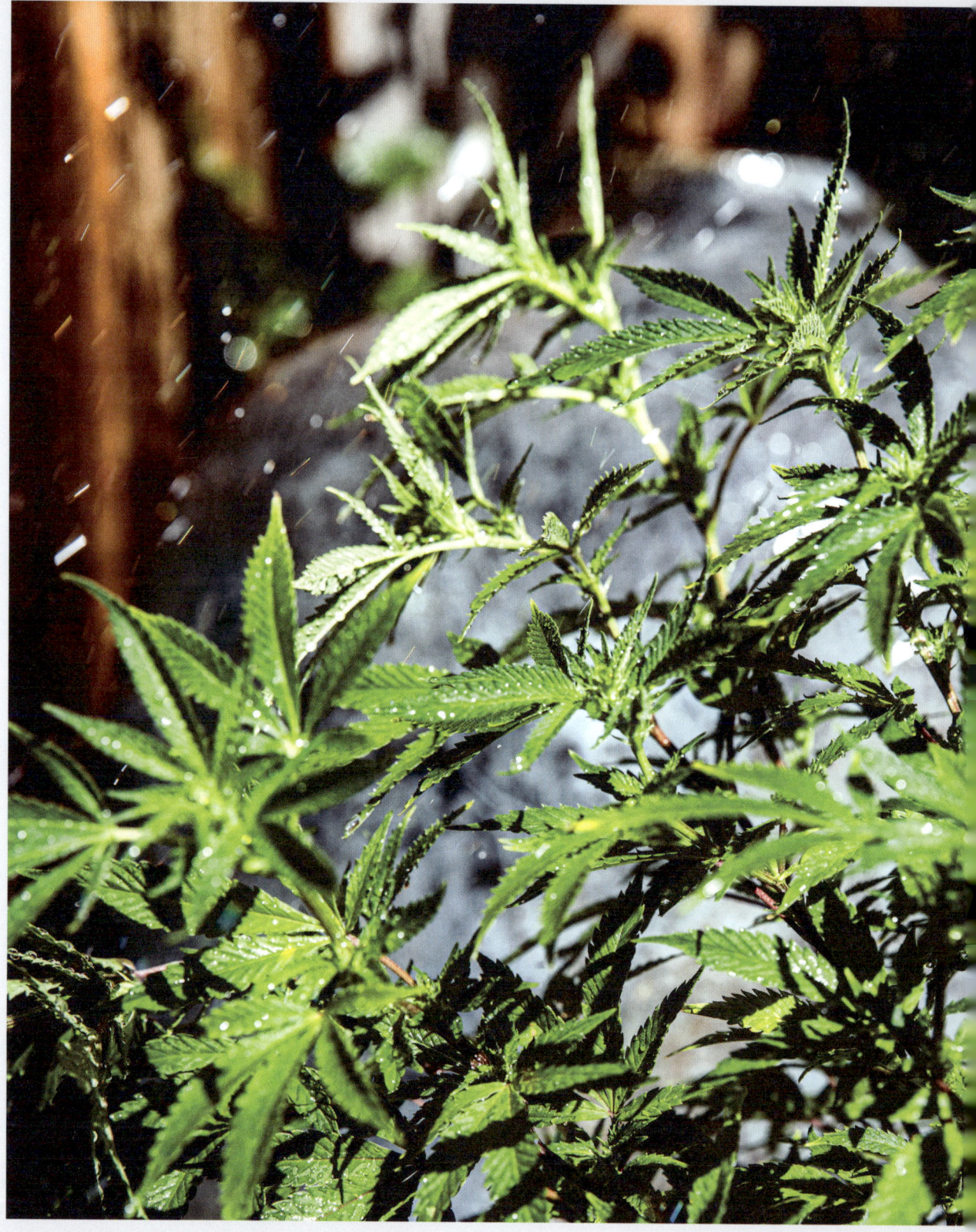

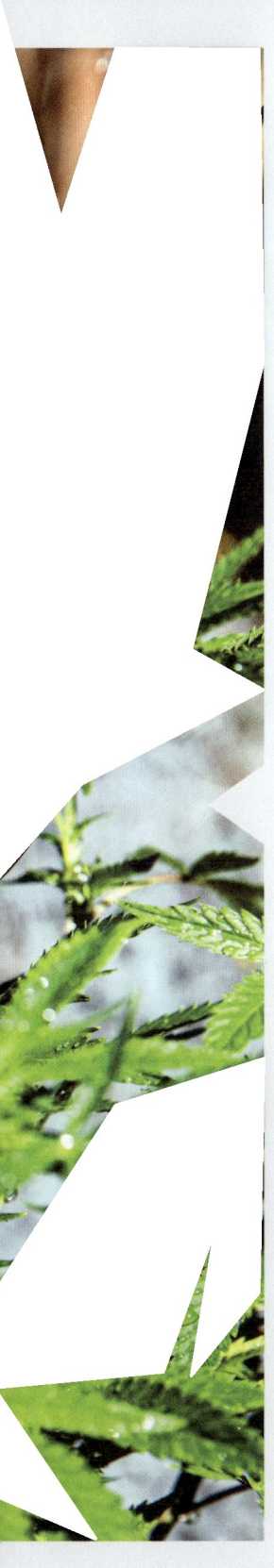

CHAPTER 3

The Four Elements:

Sun, Soil, Airflow, and Water

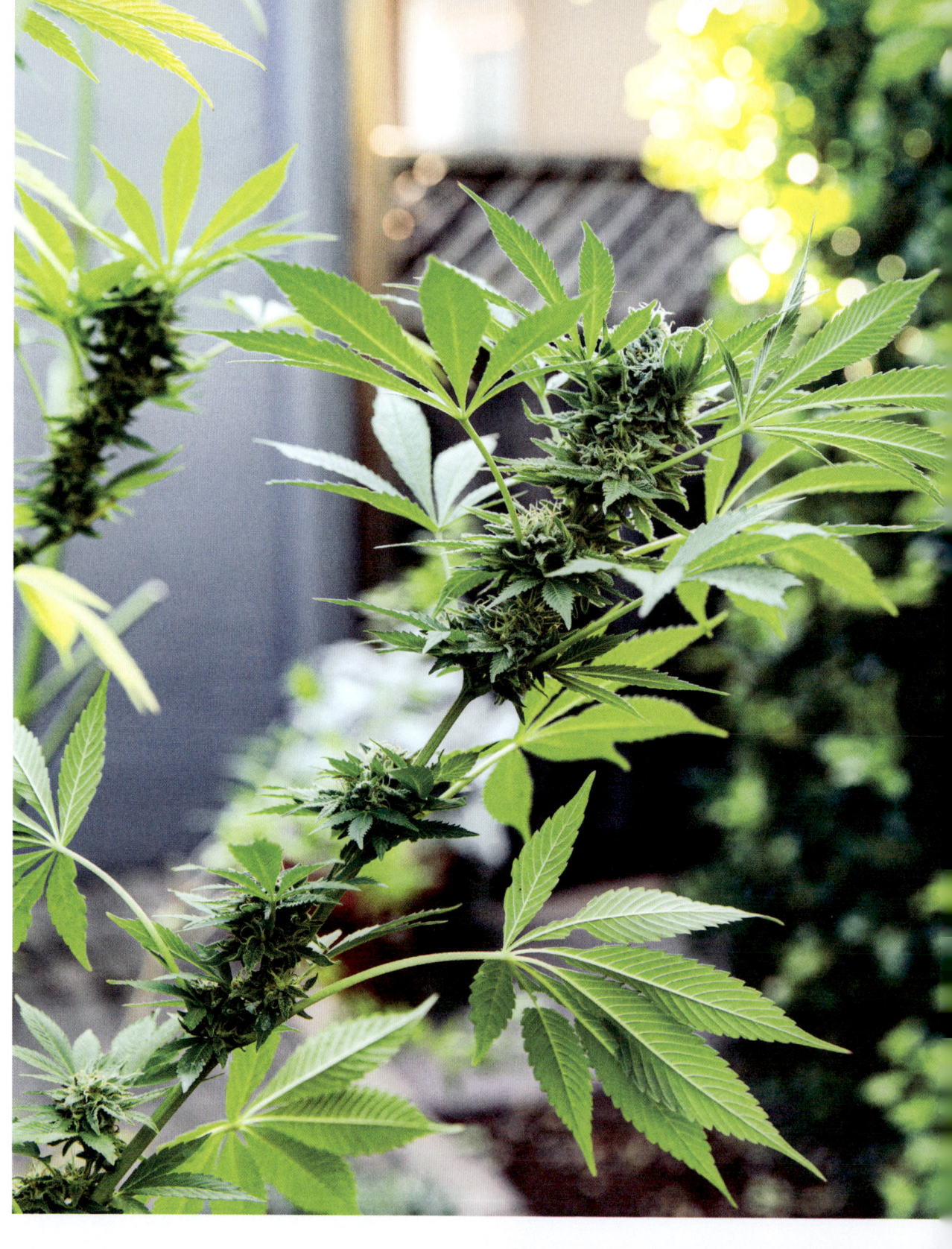

Whether you garden in a container, a raised bed, or as part of an established in-ground garden, there are priorities to keep in mind to achieve a beautiful, healthy cannabis grow. The four vital considerations as we plan our grow are sun, soil, water, and air.

SUN Sun is plant food—literally. Plants make their own food using sunshine for energy. It only makes sense that since cannabis plants are large, fast-growing annuals, they will need a lot of energy to fuel their growth. Feed your cannabis what it needs—sunlight—and it will do the rest. Cannabis needs six or more hours of direct sun per day to thrive.

If plants make their own food, then why do gardeners talk about "feeding" their plants? What exactly is plant food? Plant food is better understood as a supplement—it's all about giving plants certain nutrients that they can't manufacture out of sunshine and air. The term *fertilizer* is a more accurate one to use. There are a number of substances that plants need in order to create the hundreds of different molecules they manufacture.

The big three. The three nutrients that plants need in greatest quantity—macronutrients—are nitrogen (N), phosphorus (P), and potassium (K). If you've ever read the label on a prepared plant food, it will show these primary nutrients as three numbers, always in the order N-P-K. Nitrogen is a crucial part of chlorophyll, the vivid green molecule that allows plants to convert sun energy into sugar and cellulose. Plants also require a number of molecules in tiny amounts—micronutrients—including but not limited to magnesium, iron, calcium, zinc, boron, copper, manganese, molybdenum, and sulfur. Healthy soil, rich in decayed plant material and microbial life, provides all of these macro- and micronutrients and much more to your plant. Let nature take care of feeding your plant, and both you and your cannabis garden will be happy.

SOIL

The second of the four elements for heathy plants is soil. Cannabis is hearty and resilient—if planted in good soil. Farmer Joel Salatin describes soil this way: "Soil is life." While I differ with him on politics, I agree with him about the vital role of soil health in gardening and farming. There is more life per square foot in rich, healthy soil than anywhere else on Earth. Healthy, living soil contains up to fifty thousand microorganisms per gram of soil—an astonishing reality. There is not one soil—there are many soils—and they all have some things in common. Soil is made up of inorganic materials that are dependent on the underlying mineral types. These particles range in size from microscopically small to large rocks. These inorganic particles are the main defining characteristic of soil types and give them their names. The minerals naturally present in the inorganic portions of soil are what provide the micronutrients essential for healthy growth—but these minerals are made accessible to plants by the actions of their resident microbes. Each soil is best understood as a unique ecosystem of a vast array of microbes, fungi, insects, and animals living in a substrate (base material) of inorganic and organic material, air, and water. It is a dynamic, life-filled ecosystem into which plants plunge their roots to gain the water and micronutrients they need to grow and flourish.

Soil Fauna

Good, rich soils have abundant decayed plant matter—aka compost—as one of their key structural components. This dead and decaying plant matter is the carbon-containing portion of soil and is critical for moisture retention and for fueling the growth of its microbial life. Our soils have their own types of animals. Soil fauna refers to the animal and fungal denizens that are unique life-forms, creating and maintaining healthy soil.

Soil fauna encompass a gigantic array of life-forms, including viruses, yeasts, bacteria, fungi, protozoa, roundworms, flatworms, annelid worms, tardigrades, mites, springtails, wood lice, beetles, larvae of many insects, centipedes, millipedes, snails, slugs, ants, spiders, lizards, snakes, amphibians, and small mammals. Soil fauna aerate the soil, allowing air to penetrate below the surface and fuel aerobic respiration. Soil fauna eat and excrete a

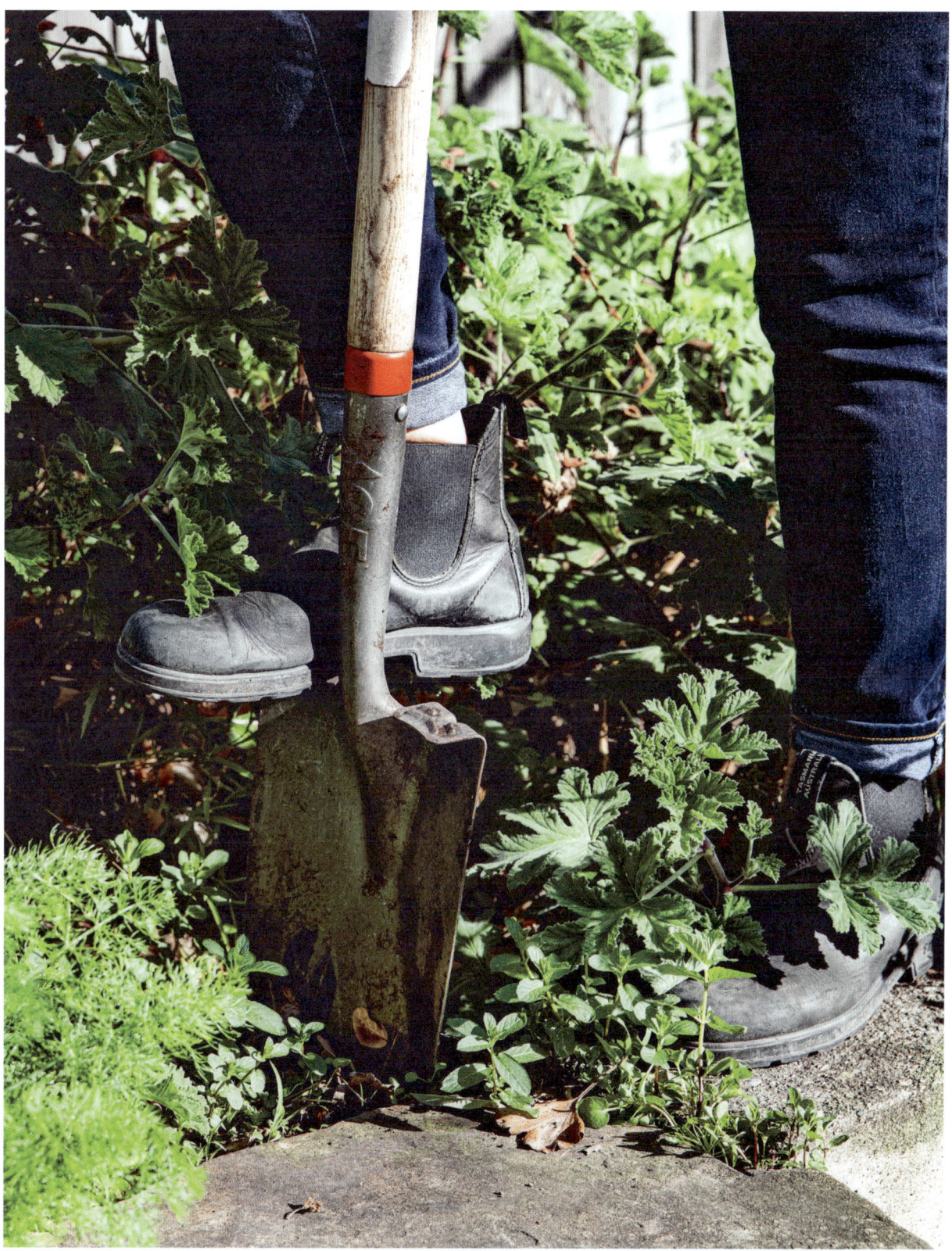

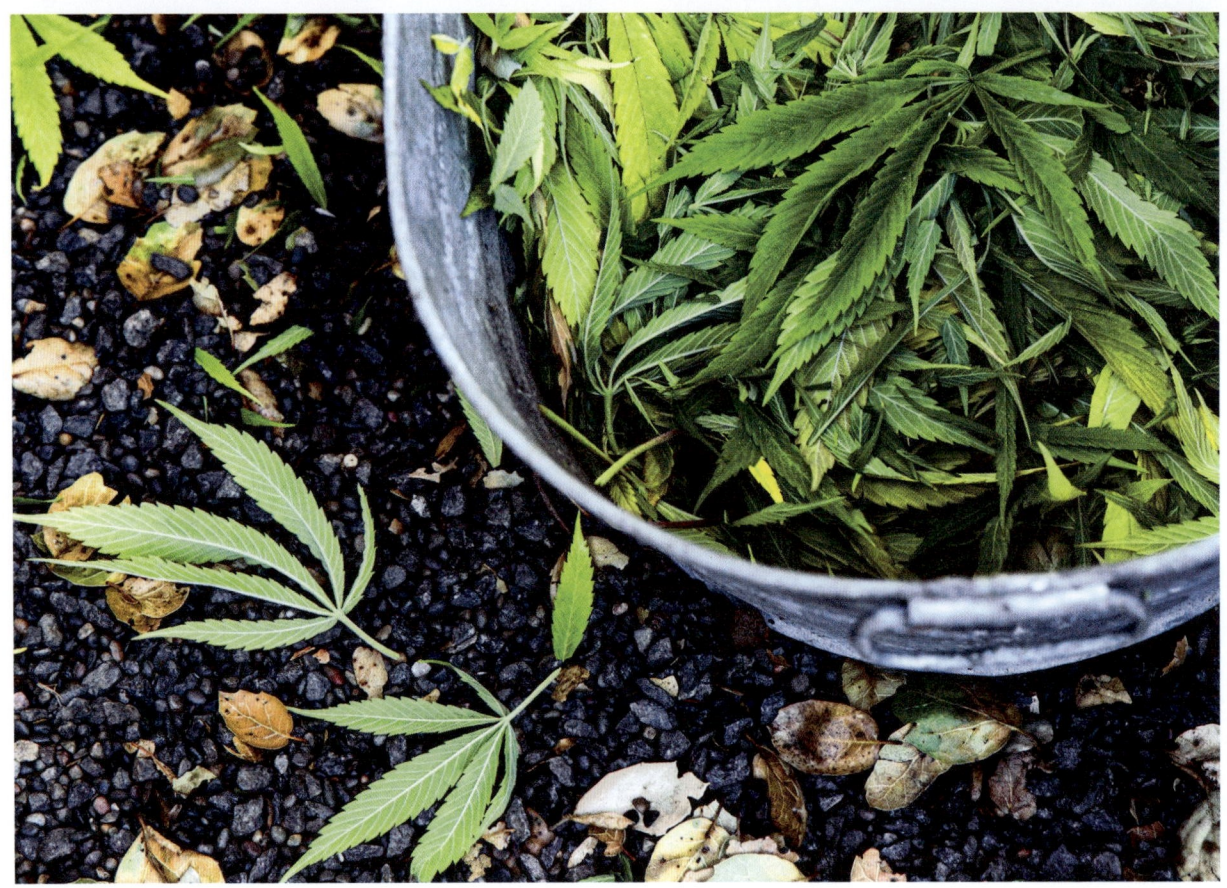

host of biologically potent substances that act to modulate the chemistry and bioavailability of micronutrients in a way that is naturally responsive to the needs of the plants living within them. Soil microbes are nature's reclamation crew. They recycle the carbon and nitrogen back into availability for other plants to use. The many types of fungi that are abundant in soils serve myriad purposes. Most plants enter into symbiotic relationships with specialized fungi to extend their root systems, while providing nutrients for the fungi.

Understand Your Soil

Healthy soil responds with a deep ability to buffer the influences of climate and moisture fluctuations and offers homeostasis (stable health) for the needs of their particular citizens. Soil is hugely important, but luckily for us, it is a largely self-organizing ecosystem. We don't have to do much—but there are a couple of ways for us to build great soils in our gardens.

Cannabis thrives in rich, well-draining, teeming-with-life soil. How do you know if your natural garden soil is good enough for your weed babies? You will need to do a little detective work. An easy place to start for those of you living in the United States is through the Master Gardener program of your local county extension office. Master Gardeners are well-trained horticulturists who volunteer in their local communities to help citizens be better gardeners. A Master Gardener will likely be able to tell you what type of soil you have, based on where you reside. You can also do a couple of quick tests to check on your soil quality. Your role as gardener is to assess the quality of your native soil and then offer it what it needs to achieve the best growing conditions. Grab a handful of your soil—how does it feel? What does it smell like? Does it clump up and then crumble or hold its shape? A good soil will hold moisture but also drain well. It should smell neutral and pleasant—not sour or stinky. Healthy natural soil will likely have worms and little crawly bugs in it—this is good. Some areas are known for good, rich bottomland soil—like the farmland in Iowa. Some soils are rich in sand and drain readily but are poor in organic material (thin sandy soil). Some soils are rich in clay and have good mineral structure but can be slow to drain when wet or pack hard when dry (clay soil).

Compost

To improve almost all soil types, there is one prescription: compost, a biologically active pile of decayed plant material. Whether you make your own compost or purchase it from your local garden center, this stuff is gardener's gold. Compost is an environmental win-win, replenishing the soil while simultaneously reducing the amount of waste in landfills. I add compost to my garden every time I plant something new—it's always helpful. The decaying plant material that makes up compost needs to be regularly added to feed the microscopic soil fauna. Nature does this all the time. Every time a leaf, twig, or a piece of dead grass falls to the ground, it slowly becomes natural compost. We interrupt this process when we tidy up our yards, inadvertently depriving our soils of the organic material nature otherwise provides. Compost is especially helpful for those of you with sandy soils because it helps these fast-draining, nutrient-poor soils hold water and become a home for happy soil microbes. Those with rocky soils similarly benefit from compost—it's pretty much a universal soil tonic.

How much compost to add is somewhat dependent on the quality of your soil. Generally, a 4-inch layer of compost dug in to a depth of at least 1 foot is an excellent start to improving thin, sandy, or clay-heavy soils. I like to dig in compost deeply in the late fall to allow the soil time to reestablish microbial activity through the winter and spring. It helps to keep in mind that you're not directly feeding your plants with compost—you're feeding your soil ecosystem, which in turn feeds your plants. Soil microbes do a far better, more nuanced job of feeding your plants than you ever could. Nature is wise. One special tip for very clay-heavy soils is to do a one-time addition of volcanic rock bits to loosen the structure of the soil. Because these rocks will break down very slowly, they won't need to be added often—only when you're expanding new garden beds.

Planting Mix

It is important to use fresh, high-quality planting mix for planting in containers, and replace the mix each growing season for best results. Many prepared planting mixes intentionally inoculate their blends with friendly soil fungus for optimal plant growth. Planting mix, also known as potting soil, that is specially formulated for growing cannabis is increasingly available at plant nurseries. I have had excellent results with E.B. Stone's Recipe 420 Potting Soil. If you have questions about the best choice of planting mix available in your area, ask for help from your local nursery.

Mulch

Mulching your living soil is another important step to bring your soil to peak condition. Mulch can be made of any dry, fluffy, organic material. A thick layer of mulch helps to retain soil moisture, and this is especially

GROWER INSIGHTS
Kate Gaudette

Kate is a farmer at Ancient Green Farm, located in mid-coast Maine. She employs hugelkultur (hill mound gardening) and regenerative farming practices, reflecting her commitment to the sustainability of the farm's products. She is a proponent of using compost teas (see page 100) to feed her soils, especially foliar teas. Kate's number one tip for cannabis gardeners is to mulch. She blankets the soil surrounding her plants with 6 to 8 inches of mulch to keep the soil temperatures and moisture levels stable, which encourages excellent soil fertility and offers optimum conditions for her cannabis and hemp plants. "Mulch, mulch, mulch!" is Kate's best advice to cannabis growers.

important for those who are growing in dry summer areas. Mulch aids soil moisture retention, keeping the root zone evenly moist and fertile, including the topmost layer, which would otherwise become dry and drive the soil microbes and fauna deeper. An added benefit for gardeners is that weeds are suppressed in mulched beds.

AIRFLOW

Airflow is important for cannabis health, so be sure to allow for good airflow around your cannabis plant, especially as it enters the final month of life and begins to flower. Proper airflow will be your best mold preventive because fungal growth occurs fastest in high-moisture environments. Air provides the carbon dioxide that plants use to combine with water and sunlight, creating carbohydrates. These carbohydrates are then used both as major building material (cellulose) and energy storage (sugars). The outdoor garden grower never has to worry about a deficit of carbon dioxide because it's provided free of charge from our atmosphere. Indoor growers often supplement the air inside their grow rooms with carbon dioxide gas to give the plants what they need—one less thing that garden growers have to concern themselves with.

Take care to plant for the future of your plant's airflow needs. The most important determiner of airflow is the space around your plant. When you find a spot in which to plant your cannabis seedling or clone, be sure to use your imagination and visualize a full-size plant. Will it have room to grow without touching another plant? And with nearby hardscaping, will your plant get crowded out by a fence or a wall? Or perhaps you need to prune surrounding mature plants to optimize airflow.

WATER

Healthy compost-rich soil is important to your plants—especially when it comes to water. All that organic matter in well-amended soil acts like a sponge, holding water near the roots and providing it as your plants need it. If you live in a climate with consistent summer rains, you may not have to provide any additional water to your cannabis, especially if it is planted in the ground. If you live in a dry summer climate, you will need to provide water to your weed plants to keep them happy. Container gardens will require watering more frequently than raised beds or in-the-ground gardens.

Tips on Watering
There are a couple tips for best watering practices, applicable to all gardens. Water in the morning to avoid loss due to evaporation in the midday heat.

Water the soil gently and slowly. Notice that I said water the soil—not water the plant. This is important for two reasons. First, cannabis leaves like being dry. They can manage well with periodic rain showers, but they are most resilient to fungal problems if their foliage is dry whenever possible. It is especially important to keep the foliage dry in muggy, humid climates. Second, watering the soil at a slow pace avoids runoff and conserves water, so it's good for the environment. For those of you with a water bill (like me), conserving water is good for the budget, too. Do not allow runoff; not only is this a wasteful practice but it also can leach nutrients from your soil and disturb the roots. There are several easy methods for watering your cannabis plants.

Soaker hose. A low-tech, flexible watering system, the soaker hose is an inexpensive, flexible porous tube that leaks water out of its entire length. It is available in a number of lengths and is very user-friendly—no special installation required. You use it by connecting your watering hose directly to the soaker hose and turning on the water for a period of time, until the soil is adequately watered. A soaker hose can be left on the ground throughout the growing season but should be taken up and stored during the winter months to preserve the life of the hose. I like to use a soaker hose to water deeply in the summer. I prefer a soaker hose to emitters or sprinklers because it won't wet the leaves and flower buds. There is some concern about the use of recycled tires in rubber soaker hoses—that they may leak toxins into the soil, which might be taken up by your cannabis plant—though the risks associated with their use is not confirmed. If you would like to err on the side of caution, consider using a food-grade polyurethane soaker hose rather than rubber.

Watering can. If you are watering planters on a deck without an outdoor spigot, I recommend investing in a high-quality gallon watering can with a wide rosette. The rosette is the perforated disk that creates fine, gentle streams of water—excellent for gently but quickly watering your soil.

Watering wand. If you hand-water your garden and have an outdoor spigot with a hose, I recommend purchasing a watering wand. If you've ever been to a plant nursery and seen the staff watering the plants, you've likely seen them use a watering wand. A watering wand is a metal tube with a wide rosette on the end, ideal for creating a gentle but high-volume stream to soak the soil without disturbing the roots. Avoid strong directional jet sprays—these are for washing driveways, not for watering plants. A gentle soak is what your soil needs.

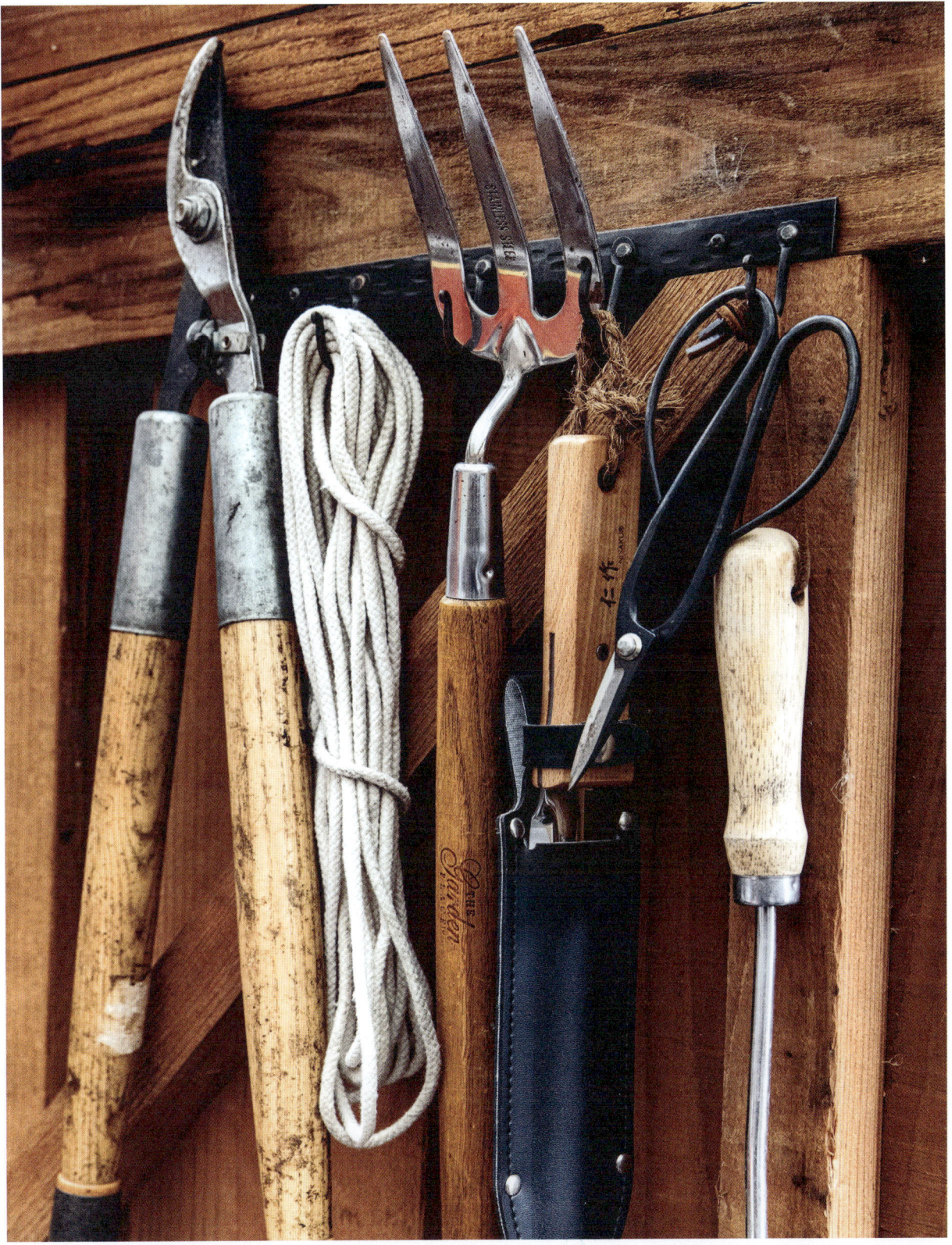

Choosing and Using Garden Tools

You don't need a lot of special equipment to be a phenomenal gardener—you can do all of your gardening with a few key pieces of equipment. I would say that about 90 percent of my gardening chores use either a spade or a pruner—these two are essential tools in my gardening kit. I recommend investing in quality tools, since they will perform well and last for years. Some pieces of equipment are more expensive, but most are quite inexpensive. Here are my go-to favorites.

SPADE. Every gardener needs a spade. A quality garden spade should be about hip height with a D-ring handle and a strong, square head. Spading the soil means to dig and turn soil. Do not confuse a spade with a shovel—they are different tools for different purposes. Shovels are fine for moving loose material but not for turning the soil. Spades do not need to be costly. In fact, over the years of trying out different spades, my favorite is an inexpensive model from the local hardware store.

PRUNING SHEARS. This handheld tool is essential for any gardener. I am a fan of Felco tools; they are costly but last for decades. There are two main types of pruning shears: bypass shears for live branches and anvil shears for dead branches. Well-made pruning shears are available in several sizes for the ideal fit, configured for right-hand or left-hand use, and available in different designs. They are a worthy investment. On a personal note, I have used one pair of little Felco 6 pruning shears for twenty-five years, and they are still going strong. I love how their petite size fits so snugly in my hand, but they can still cut through slender branches with ease.

TROWEL. A hand trowel is very handy for planting and digging up weeds. These are inexpensive, readily available, and come in many colors and styles. I recommend choosing a trowel with a strong, stiff body and a handle that feels comfortable and secure in your hand. My favorite trowel is actually a Japanese garden knife called a hori-hori. The hori-hori is fabulously efficient at digging out weeds and makes quick work of loosening soil for planting out seedlings. "Hori-hori" is onomatopoeia for "dig-dig."

NEJIRI SCRAPER. This small lightweight hand tool is composed of a wooden handle, a metal neck, and topped with a sharp steel triangular head. This left- or right-handed scraper is my go-to for fine weeding, especially for newly sprouted seeds. Inexpensive but effective, this tool is available at well-stocked garden stores, Japanese tool stores, and online.

GLOVES. Garden gloves are a key part of my gardening tool set because they offer protection to keep my best garden tool—my hands—in top shape. I love getting my bare hands in the soil. They take a beating, though, with constant exposure to the soil and plants. I keep two types of gloves on hand at all times. My favorite is a pair of nitrile-dipped knit gloves. There are lots of brands from which to choose, and they are inexpensive. Make sure you choose the right size for your hands. They should provide a nice grip, feel comfortable, and, best of all, be machine washable. The other pair of gloves I have are thin, close-fitting gardening gloves for fine weeding or baby seedling transfers. I like these when I need protection from wet soils but need a responsive feel for more delicate gardening tasks.

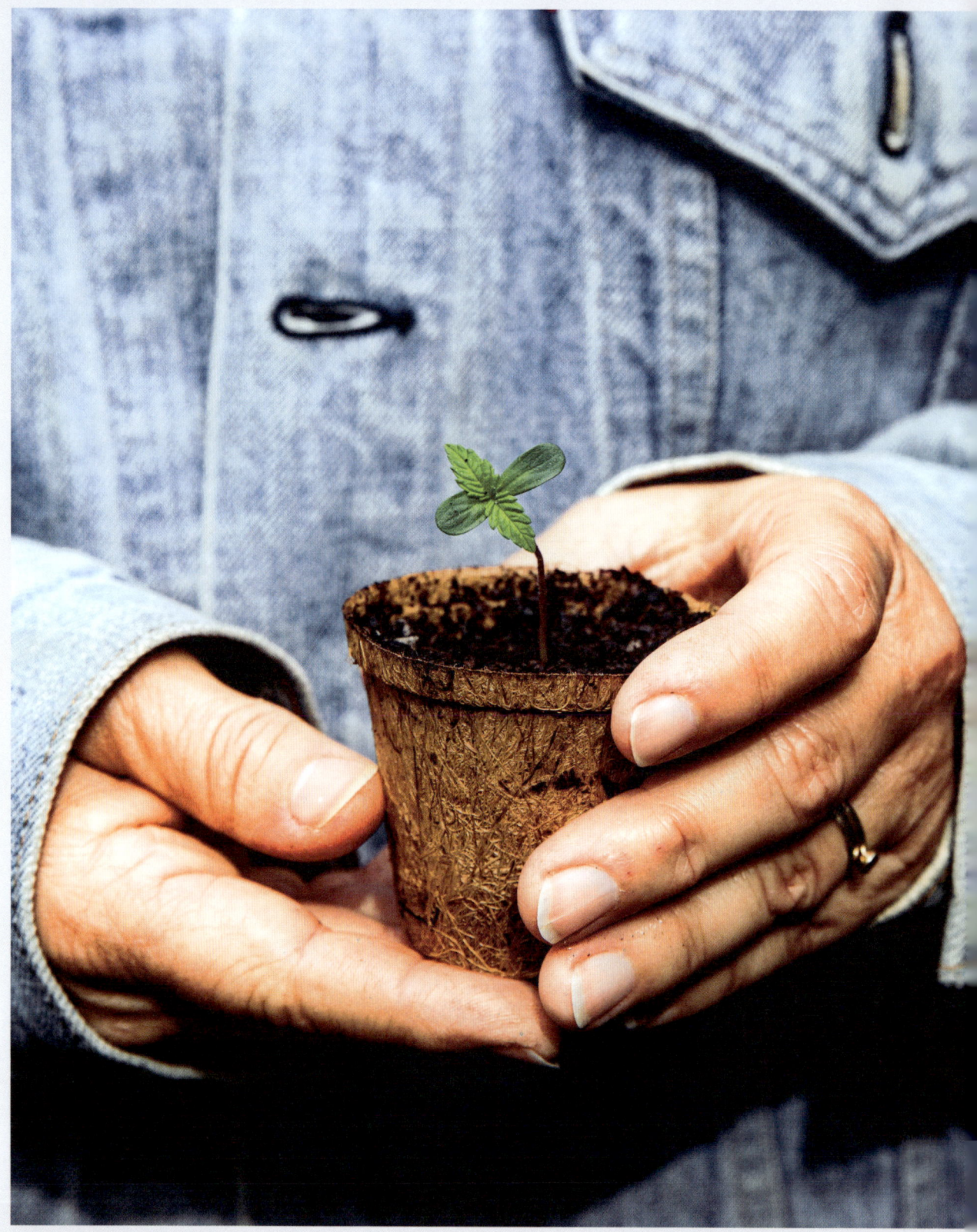

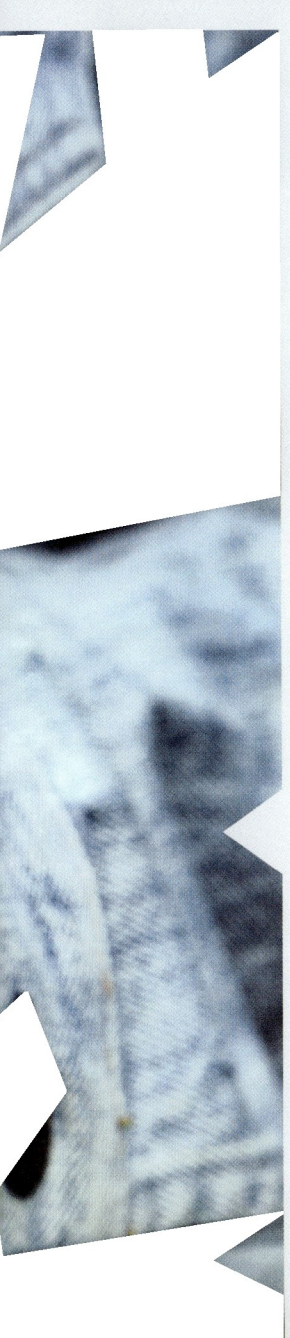

CHAPTER 4

The Vegetative Stage:

From Seed to Teen

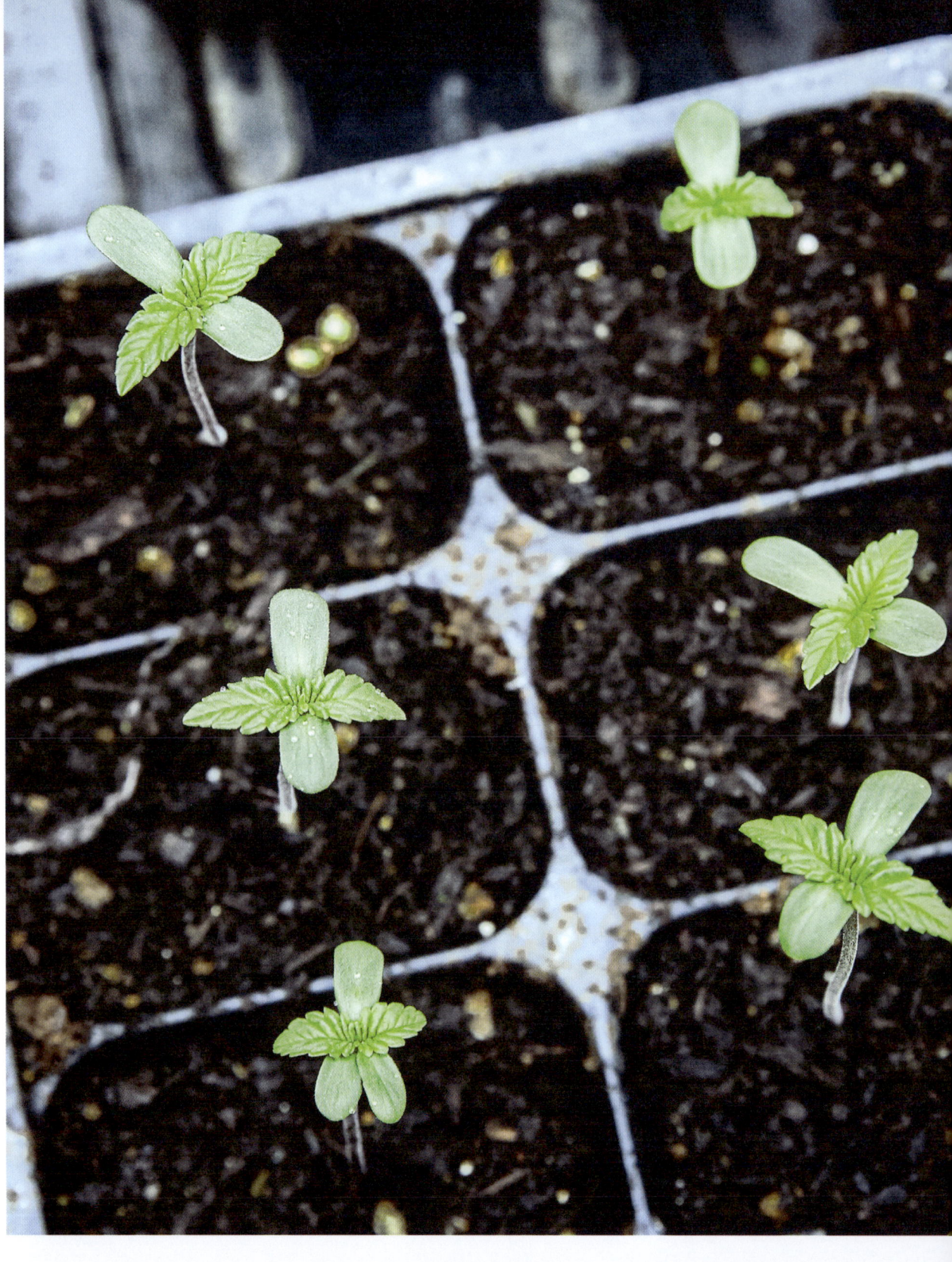

Let's dig into how to grow your own cannabis victory garden. We'll start at the beginning, with a discussion of whether to plant a seed or a clone, then move on to step-by-step growing instructions to take your cannabis plant through the first portion of life: the vegetative stage. The use of the term *vegetative stage* is common in the cannabis growing community, especially so with indoor growers who use artificial lights to simulate sunlight and its seasonal fluctuations. As this magnificent plant becomes mainstreamed in gardening culture, I anticipate that we'll drop the use of the term altogether. Its one usefulness for the outdoor gardener is that the plant has some tailored needs during each season, and it helps to think of the plant in discrete stages to optimize gardening tasks. The vegetative—or veg—stage is the time when your cannabis goes from seed or clone to a lush full-grown plant, poised to begin flowering. This stage is filled with exuberant growth—taking a tiny seed to a huge plant in just a few months.

A LITTLE BIT OF BOTANY

Before we dive into how to grow your cannabis, let's learn a little botany. Flowers are the sex organs of flowering plants—but not all flowers are the same. Some plants produce perfect or complete flowers—meaning that each of their flowers has both male and female parts and is therefore capable of self-pollination. Some plants—monoecious plants—produce imperfect flowers, meaning that there are two different types of flowers, male (pollen-producing) and female (seed-producing) flowers on the same plant. Another type of plant—the dioecious plant—produces either male *or* female flowers on different plants. Cannabis is a dioecious plant. Nearly all dioecious plants are perennials and include several familiar gardening plants, including holly, ginkgo, maple, pistachio, bay laurel, mulberry, and hops, to name a few. Cannabis is a rare one—it is an *annual* dioecious plant. There are two sexes of cannabis, female and male. Female plants make only female flowers, and male plants produce only male flowers. Seeds form when male cannabis pollen falls on female flowers. This is important for any cannabis grower to know, because it is the unfertilized female flowers we are after. The exception to this is the grower who wants cannabis seeds for next year's grow (see page 96).

Unfertilized female flower buds are sparkly with trichomes, and these trichomes are what create almost all of the plant's cannabinoids and terpenes that are so helpful to our bodies and minds. From the plant's perspective, the resins within the trichomes are what help trap pollen and ward off insect damage. As soon as the plant is pollinated, the female cannabis plant turns its attention and energy to seed production—not what we usually want from our grow.

THE ROAD TO SUCCESS

Cannabis gardeners will make a key decision at the start of the growing season. Will I plant a clone or a seed? Which one is best for my garden? Both can work—but there are benefits and drawbacks to each. Let's explore the pros and cons of growing from clone or seed.

The Pros and Cons of Clones

If you've had experience with indoor cannabis growing, you may be familiar with clones. The term *clone* is a bit of a misnomer, but it's what is commonly used in the cannabis trade. Clones are best thought of as an extension of the mother plant, rather than as a different—albeit genetically identical—plant. Clones are made by removing a small section of a lateral branch tip from a mother plant, trimming off the lower leaves, and placing the cut end of the branch tip into growth medium. Common growth mediums for rooting these cuttings are rock wool and coconut coir.

Several days after being placed in its growth medium, the cutting puts out roots—called adventitious roots—and then begins to grow as a separate plant. These rooted cuttings are then offered for sale at dispensaries and are ready to be hardened off and planted in your garden. While dedicated home growers can produce their own cuttings, most of us will purchase clones from local dispensaries.

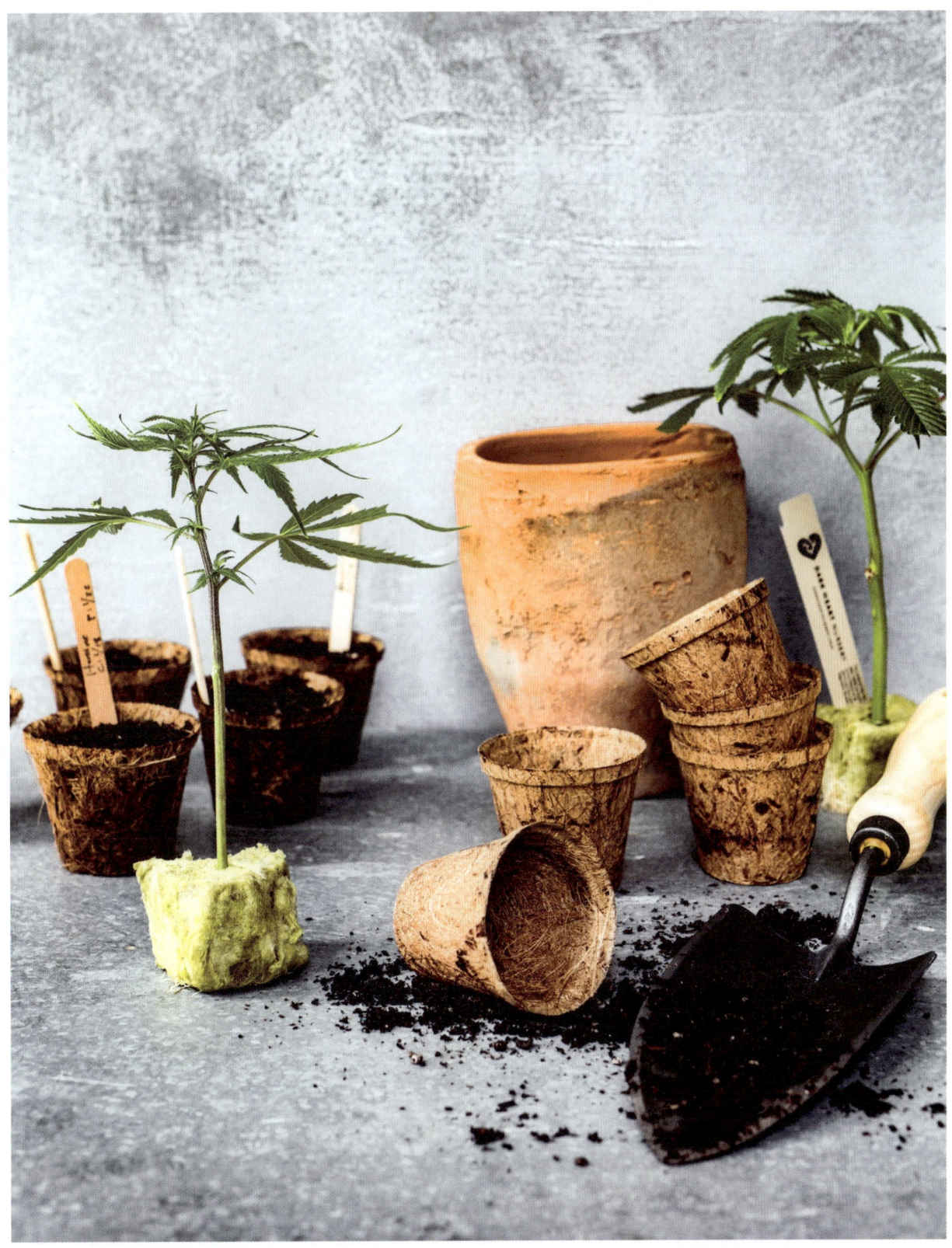

Rooted cuttings/clones are not the same as tissue culture cannabis plants, which are true clones. Tissue culture is a more technical horticulture technique that emerged commercially in the 1950s and is currently applied to high-value food and floriculture crops, where specific genetics are of prime importance. This is a technique that takes a tiny portion of a plant and incubates it in a petri dish on a special growth medium, resulting in a true genetic clone, complete with a taproot. Tissue culture cannabis plants are so far not available to non-commercial growers but may be in the future, since cannabis legalization nationwide encourages scale and the investment money that follows. For the purposes of this book, the term *clone* will refer to a rooted cutting—not a tissue culture plant.

Clones are a great choice for container gardening and an appropriate choice for raised beds. Because they are selected from established mother plants, you can rest assured that the clone will be female and a well-known cultivar. For those of you seeking a specific cultivar of cannabis, clones offer reliable and predictable results from your harvest. Growing from clones gives you a head start on the growing season and minimizes your front-end propagation efforts. Just plop the little clone in your prepared soil, water, and enjoy.

The downside to growing with clones is that they are not complete plants—they do not have taproots. As a result, they will not get as large and robust as a seedling grown plant. There are fewer cultivars of clones than cannabis seeds available to home cannabis gardeners, though those available as clones are typically user favorites. Clones have a small risk of transmitting disease from the grower to your garden, but if you choose a well-grown product from a reputable propagator, this risk is minimized. Because cannabis is a fast-growing plant, clones are perishable, so they need to be planted soon after bringing them home from the dispensary.

The Pros and Cons of Seeds

Seed-grown cannabis is an excellent choice for planting in the ground or in raised beds. There is an overwhelming variety of cannabis cultivar seeds from which to choose, and their names are awesomely creative, though sometimes more fun than descriptive. Cannabis seeds are easy to sprout and grow vigorously. But there's a catch. As I discussed earlier, cannabis comes in two sexes—and you can't tell from looking at them which seeds are female and which ones are male. Lucky for us, cannabis growers are clever and have figured out how to produce all-female cannabis seeds that are called, for obvious reasons, feminized seeds (see Sources, page 178).

Dan Grace

I recently had the privilege of visiting the grow room of Dark Heart Nursery. Dan Grace, its CEO, led us through the facility and described their cannabis horticultural practices. My favorite part of the tour was when we viewed the nursery's inner sanctum, where they tend their treasured collection of mother plants—the mature female plants from which they take cuttings to create clones. Since cannabis is an annual plant, they have to use special lighting to convince these lovely ladies that it's always summer so they stay in the veg stage. Seeing Dan's well-run operation made me so appreciative of the care and passion that is needed to keep the cannabis plants safe and healthy for gardeners and commercial growers alike.

Feminized seeds are created by treating a high-quality cannabis female with silver thiosulfate or gibberellic acid to force a branch section of the female plant to produce male pollen-containing flowers. These male flowers still have only female chromosomes. They self-cross the pollen to the female flowers on the same plant or on another female plant and harvest the resulting all-female seeds. By choosing feminized seeds, you are sure to get a female plant. This is a great choice for those of you who want a tall, vigorous plant but don't want to risk the space or waste your time waiting to find out if your plant is a boy or a girl. The only drawback is that not all cultivars are available in feminized form. If you choose to grow from regular seeds (that is, from seeds as nature makes them), you will need to sex your plants as the preflowers emerge. (See page 79 for more information on how to sex your plants.) Rest assured—cannabis is such a happy, vigorous garden plant that you will get great results from either feminized seed or regular seed.

A Cultivar by Any Other Name

The very concept of cultivar (or strain, the term used in the commercial cannabis community) is one of some controversy in the cannabis world. Two cannabis seed packs sold under the same name may not, in fact, *be* the same. Some cultivars may be nearly identical to the original, but some may be really different. Why is that? Because each cannabis seedling is

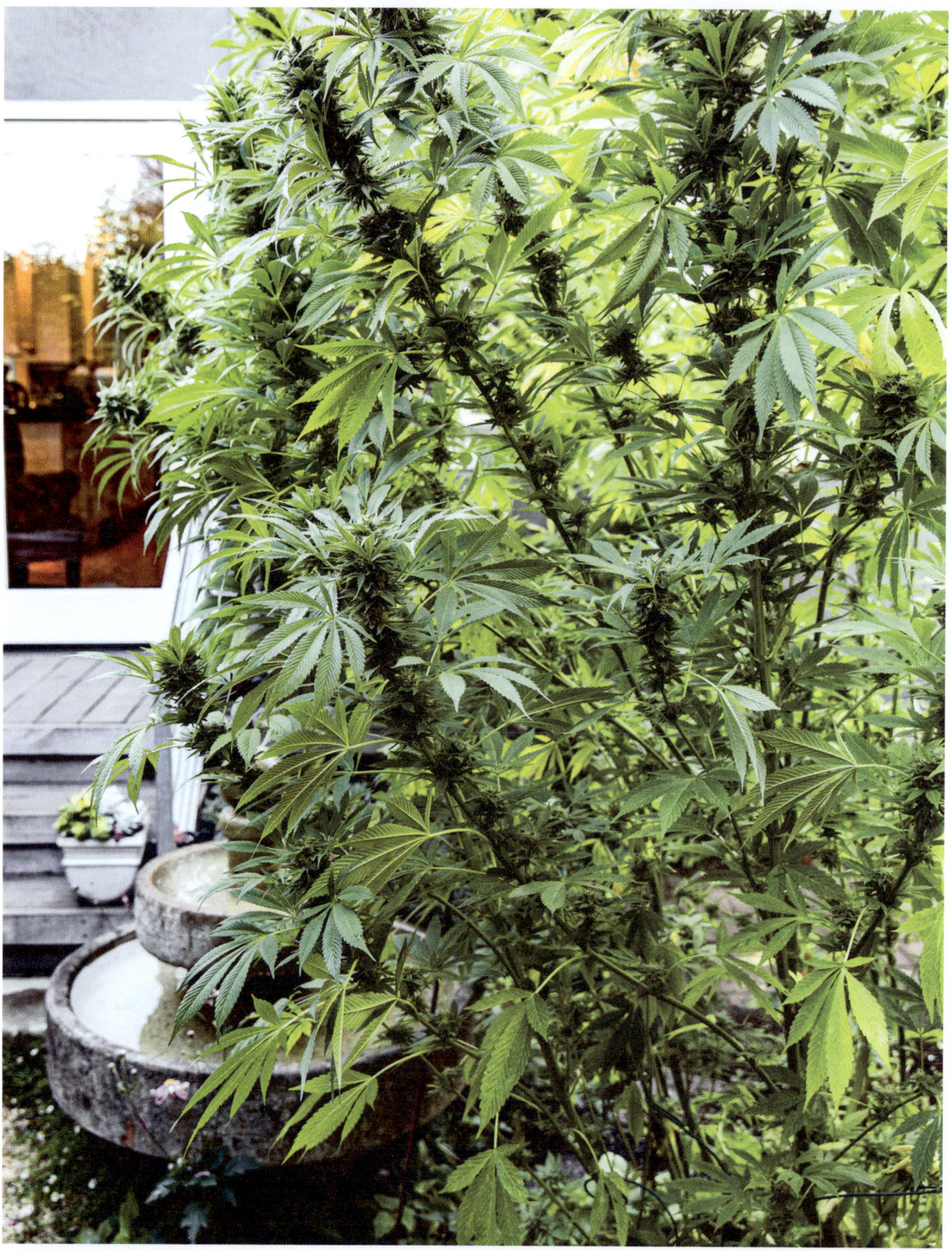

genetically unique—just as people are. But if every cannabis seedling has a unique genetic makeup, how can any nonclone type of cannabis be a true cultivar type of cannabis? When is a Blue Dream seedling Blue Dream, and when is it better understood to be something else? This is both a marketing issue and a reality check. While no two seedlings are ever exactly alike, they can become generationally alike enough to retain a readily identifiable characteristic—and thus remain true to type. In the heirloom gardening world, it's well known that it takes many generations for a set of plant traits to stabilize, or exhibit consistency, year after year. The same is true for cannabis.

You may encounter a seed description as F1 in a cannabis seed catalog. This nomenclature will be familiar to the experienced vegetable gardener—and it is important to understand this as it relates to notions of hybrid vigor and seed stability. Let's say that a grower has two cannabis cultivars that are each really great but are different from each other. Maybe the female is tall, smells lemony, and is super potent with THC. The male is stockier, smells like lavender, and offers high CBD. Sounds like an interesting combo, right? So, what would happen if you crossbred these two? The first generation of seedlings—the F1 generation—would combine some of the traits of each parent and would all be relatively consistent with each other. This is why many plant breeders offer F1 seeds for sale. It's because they get vigorous, relatively predictable seedlings from this first generation of crosses. The strength of this first generation is well known in the horticulture world—it's called hybrid vigor. Now, take two of these seedlings—F1 × F1—cross them, and you get the grandchildren of the original two. This is the F2 generation. This generation will likely exhibit a lot of diversity, even if the two F1 plant parents were pretty similar. This seed line will need to be recrossed for many more generations before becoming stable. When you encounter the term *stabilized* in cannabis seed catalogs, you can rest assured that you are going to get predictable results from the plant.

Autos: Cannabis for Short Seasons and Small Spaces

Cannabis is photoperiod sensitive, as are many plants that originated in a natural temperate zone. This means that cannabis plants know to start blooming when nighttime darkness is twelve hours or more. For subtropical and temperate zones, we can grow many types of cannabis. But for those growers in zones that have strong seasonal changes in light, cannabis can be a challenge to grow outside, because by the time the nights lengthen enough to trigger flowering, the cold weather of fall kills the plants before they mature.

But there is good news. There is a newer type of cannabis on the market, the auto-flowering cannabis, or "auto" for short. These are unique cannabis plants in that they are day-neutral—triggered to flower in a specific amount of time after sprouting, regardless of the amount of light or daylight they receive. Autos are the result of crossing existing good-quality medicinal/drug cultivars with a cannabis subspecies called *Cannabis sativa ruderalis,* or "ruderalis." The ruderalis subspecies of cannabis originated in the brief growing season, harsh winter area of central Asia, where the plants couldn't depend on the changes in season to trigger flowering early enough for them to finish before they were killed by a freeze. Winter came too quickly for these photoperiod plants to reliably set seed.

Auto-flowers are helpful for those who live in northerly climates with short growing seasons, like Alaska, and for those in true tropical climates, like Hawaii. Auto-flowers bloom reliably in a short growing period, so they are ideal for getting in two crops per year in a warm tropical area. The opposite condition occurs in far northerly or short summer climates, including the northern US East Coast, the upper Midwest, and the high-latitude growing areas like Juneau, Alaska, where there is a short but intense growing season with super-long summer days. Auto-flowers are perfect for these areas because the plants can reliably mature before the first killing frosts of autumn happen.

Another benefit for auto-flower growers is the relatively compact size of the plant. This makes autos ideal for growers with a small gardening space. Auto-flowering cannabis will grow anywhere—so for those of you in prime cannabis growing territory but who want something new, try an auto-flower.

PLANNING IS KEY

Winter is a gardener's dreaming time—an opportunity to reflect on last season's joys and make note of improvements to put in place going forward. This is the time to visit cannabis growers' websites, research what's available on the market, see what's new since last year, and make some strategic purchases. (To help you choose the right cannabis for you and your garden, see chapter 1.)

Starting from Seed

For those of you planting seedlings, your growing season begins by securing some cannabis seeds.

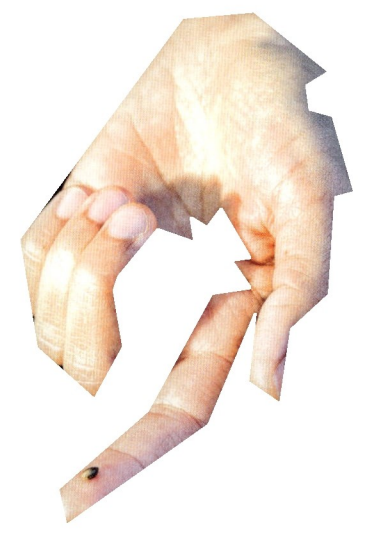

Choosing which type of seed. Start by identifying the general type of cannabis you want in terms of its cannabinoid/terpene profile (see pages 20–21). Go through this list and make sure that these seeds are suitable for your garden's climate and space limitations, then decide if you want regular or feminized seed. These few decisions will focus your search and help you quickly short-list a great selection of seeds to pursue.

Choosing how many seeds to buy. As for how many seeds to purchase, keep in mind two things. First, consider how many plants you both have room for and are legally allowed to grow, then purchase that number of feminized seeds; double this number for regular seed. While good-quality fresh cannabis seeds have a high germination rate, you may want to purchase a few extra seeds for insurance against seed failure—or to give away to a neighbor for their grow.

Choosing where to buy seeds. It can be a little overwhelming to choose where to purchase your cannabis seeds. You can purchase seeds at dispensaries or through the mail. There are also many cannabis seed sellers online. If you live close to a good dispensary that sells seed, start there. You can learn a lot from the budtenders about which breeders' seeds get good reviews. The main drawback of getting your seed from a dispensary is limited selection. If you purchase from an online source, stick with breeders with a strong track record of high-quality plants. Since legally purchasing cannabis seed on the open market is still new and quickly gaining traction, the availability of seed at any given time is hit or miss. One more thing to note—cannabis seeds can be quite expensive compared to just about any other plant seed on the market. When you consider the value of a cannabis crop—up to a pound of dried bud from one seed—the cost falls into perspective. See Sources (page 178) for a list of reputable cannabis seed sellers. Since the cannabis industry is constantly changing, this list will likely be out of date soon after the book's publication. I recommend using this list as a start to your research, then continue your research at local dispensaries and online.

Growing from Clones

For those of you who will be growing from clones, the research to acquire clones is pretty much the same as it is for seeds. Start with what health impacts you want, identify which plants will grow well in your climate and space, and then go shopping at your local dispensary to find the best

> ## In my garden . . .

With so many choices of cannabis seed, it can be tough to decide what to grow. Here's how I whittled down my list last year. I decided to grow a cannabis cultivar with equal expression of CBD:THC, and fresh lemony terpenes. I wanted to grow from feminized seed, as this eliminates the male plants. This narrowed down my search considerably, and I ended up purchasing Pennywise 1:1 feminized seed. (A great choice for me and my garden, BTW!) I looked online and at local dispensaries and located a five-pack of these seeds for $60. I sprouted and grew four of these seeds (I lost one seed to my gravel, sadly) and gave two baby seedlings to a friend. I planted the two remaining seedlings in my garden along with three other varieties.

clones for you and your garden. Some growers will ship clones through the mail, so this may expand your choices.

Seeking the Unusual

For maverick gardeners (you know who you are), cannabis is about to be your new favorite plant. There are some cool cannabis oddball strains that produce unusual-looking leaves or exhibit weird growth patterns. These plants are for gardeners seeking novelty—rather than a particular medical impact—although these plants can have nice cannabinoids and terpenes. If you have room in your garden and want something fabulous to show off to your cannabis-savvy friends, try one of the unusual strains, such as Freak Show, Dr. Grinspoon, or Australian Bastard—this list is sure to grow as breeders get more creative. No matter what variety of cannabis you choose to grow, you will be richly rewarded.

IT'S TIME TO PLANT You've chosen a great strain of cannabis for your body and your garden, purchased your seeds, and selected the perfect site in your garden—either a container, a raised bed, or in the ground. Your soil is well amended with compost and spring has arrived. Three weeks before you know that you can safely plant your baby cannabis plants outside (this will be different for each climate zone), it's time to crack your seeds.

How to Crack Seeds

Cracking seeds simply means hydrating the seeds in warm water until they swell and begin to push their radicles through the seed coat. You can skip this step and proceed directly to sowing the seeds in your seedling tray, but I recommend cracking your seeds prior to planting in soil the first time you grow weed. Why? Because it's pure joy to witness those baby cannabis plants come to life.

Seeds are one of the most amazing things in nature. A cannabis seed is composed of a few parts: the seed coat, food stores, and a living embryonic plant. If you purchase cannabis seeds from a reputable grower, all of your seeds should sprout and grow well. While properly stored cannabis seeds can remain viable for decades, their germination rate decreases over time, so it's best to plant seeds from the past season or two. Cannabis seeds are oval and about 3 to 4 millimeters in length, with smooth seed coats. The seed colors typically show muted coloration including tan, olive green, gray, and brown and are mottled or uniform in tone. Although a few cannabis seeds are naturally pale at maturity, most are darker in color. Avoid purchasing very pale seeds or seeds that aren't hard and dense with smooth seed coats, as these seeds were probably immature at harvest and unlikely to germinate and grow.

To crack the seeds, place your seeds in a small container and cover with ½ inch or so of room-temperature tap water. The seeds will likely float on top of the water. Give them a little poke to relieve the naturally occurring surface tension of the water, then allow them to soak for several hours, until the seeds absorb enough water to fully hydrate and a few begin to sink to the bottom of the container. Moisten a paper towel or a clean, soft cotton dish towel and place it on a plate or shallow dish. Enfold the moist towel over the cannabis seeds to provide even moisture. Keep the towel and seeds evenly moist for a day or two, checking once or twice a day until you see evidence of a baby root emerging from the seed coat. When most of the seeds have cracked, it's time to transfer them to their nursery.

Sowing the Seeds

Sow the seeds into a small divided seedling tray filled with high-quality, finely textured potting soil. You can also use an egg carton for the seedling sprouting stage. There are good-quality commercial sprouting mixes available in nurseries. Although there are some who insist that the seedling mix needs to be sterilized, I have had good success with regular planting mix. Poke a little hole in the center of each division about ¼ inch deep. Plop one cracked seed into each hole, then gently cover the seed with soil. Cannabis seeds are eager sprouters, so you should expect most, if not all, of your cracked seeds to sprout soon after being planted. Older seeds (more than one year old) will be slower to sprout. If you have a lone seed or two that doesn't crack but the rest are cracked, go ahead and plant them to see if they sprout. Seeds are living beings, each with its own little clock.

Keep the soil in the seedling tray evenly moist—being careful not to allow any standing water to remain after moistening or let the soil become too dry. This step will require daily monitoring for ideal results, since these tiny soil blocks can dry quickly if exposed to the warmth of a sunny windowsill. Many seedling trays come with a clear domed top to trap moisture, which is helpful to use while the seeds are not yet sprouted. After the seeds begin to emerge from the soil, I suggest leaving the seedling tray exposed to fresh air; this will help prevent any harmful fungal attack of your baby seedlings. Keep the temperature for your seed tray between 75°F and 80°F while they're sprouting and maintain high (70 percent) humidity.

Developing a root system. Now it's time for the magic to happen. The little seeds will be continuing their miraculous transformation under the surface of the soil. Remember the little white radicle that emerged from the seed when you cracked it? This now becomes the systemic root system, including the all-important taproot of your cannabis plant. This little taproot will eventually grow deep and strong in the soil, allowing this tiny seedling to grow to full potential in a matter of months—perhaps 13 or more feet tall. One by one your seedlings will then push their seed leaves—known as cotyledons—up and out of the soil, shedding the seed coat and widening into a tiny two-leaved plant. At this point, these little babies need light to fuel their rapid growth. If you happen to live in a seedling-friendly climate, you can sprout the seeds outside.

Let there be light. Even in the mild and easy weather of the Bay Area, I prefer the consistency of indoor lighting for the first couple weeks of life, especially when I sprout seeds in early spring. I use a T-5 fluorescent light hung a few inches from the top of the soil surface of the seedling tray. This is an energy-efficient, cool-temperature light that provides the spectrum for seedlings to thrive. I keep this light on for eighteen hours per day as the seeds are sprouting, although it's also fine to keep it on for twenty-four hours per day. Cannabis seedlings grow fast and can stretch, or develop long spindly stems, if not given strong light right when they sprout. Your baby seedlings like moderate temperatures of 65°F to 80°F. Remember that little taproot? It is critical for your plant, and your cannabis plant can't replace it in case it gets broken or damaged. Keep this in mind as you

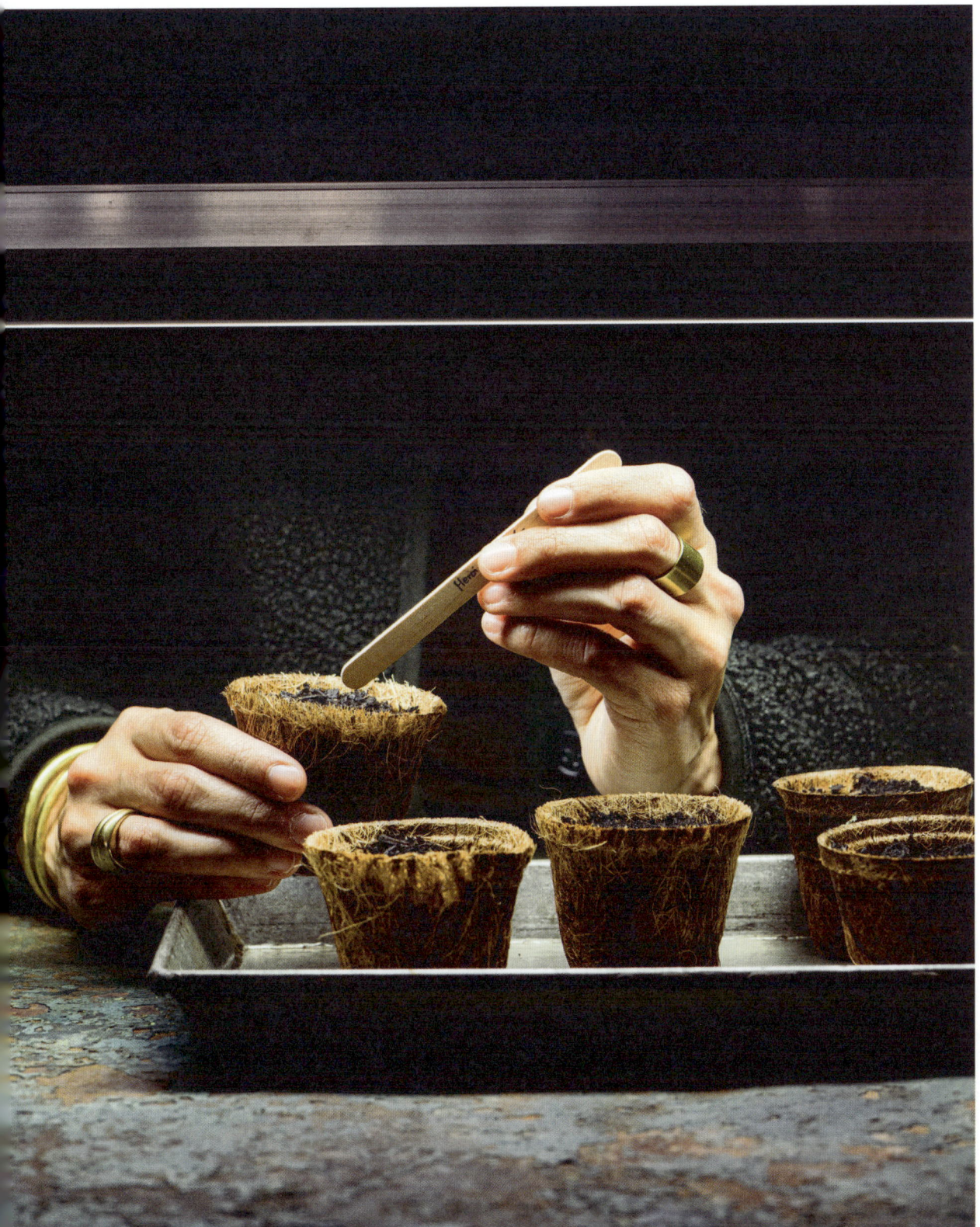

nurture your little plants and focus on giving them enough space to grow into healthy, vigorous plants.

The taproot is continuing to grow as the tiny seedlings develop their second and third sets of leaves. You'll notice that the first two "leaves" that the cannabis plant makes are rounded and relatively succulent. These seed leaves, or cotyledons, started as the two halves of the seed. They undergo an amazing transformation as they emerge from the soil surface. They emerge a beige color but quickly turn bright green, begin to photosynthesize, and grow larger. The next little set of leaves—and for cannabis there are always two that emerge at once—are the first "true" leaves and will look different from the cotyledons. These true leaves will be ruffled, pointed, and ribbed, and the next set of true leaves will be bigger still.

From Baby to Toddler

Once the seedlings have one or two sets of true leaves, it's time for them to get a bigger home. At this point, transfer each seedling to a plastic or paper quart-size pot filled with high-quality planting mix; this is where they will stay for about three weeks. I like to use pots that are deeper than wide for this time in the cannabis's life. I find that this allows the taproot to grow nice and straight. Since your cannabis babies are going to be potted in these quart-size pots for only a few weeks, a sturdy brown paper bag can

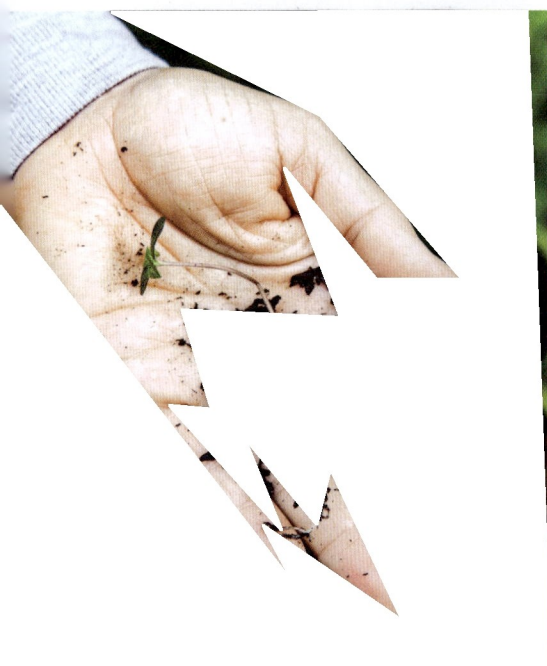

also be a fine option as a temporary pot. When it is time to put your growing cannabis plant in its permanent location, you can place the whole bag directly into its final home. The brown paper quickly biodegrades. You could—if needed—plant the young seedlings directly into the large final growing spot. This entails more risk of failure, but if you have extra seedlings and are willing to take a chance on less-than-ideal conditions, go for it. But for the best conditions, I recommend sending your baby seedlings to "nursery school" before planting them directly outside.

During this toddler stage, you will need to give your cannabis toddlers sunshine or appropriate artificial light for fourteen or more hours per day. Keep the soil evenly moist and provide gentle airflow to ward off harmful fungal growth, especially if you are growing the young cannabis plants inside. Cannabis is a vigorous grower, and once it gets off to a healthy start, it grows quickly. I love this stage in the cannabis gardening journey. Spring is such a deliciously hopeful season, and cannabis plants are exuberant expressions of this season of green.

Test for sex. A special note for those of you growing from regular (non-feminized) seed. You will have two opportunities to sex your plants, and one of them is early—before you plant in the ground or in a large pot. The "early sexing method" genetically tests a tiny portion of your baby plants for gender. Phylos BioScience offers a sexing test for your plants that costs about $60 for four plant tests (see Sources, page 178). This is a by-mail test that offers very early results to help you know what sex your plants are. If you have space for only a few plants, it can be especially disappointing to have to pull up male plants later in the season. I appreciate knowing the sex of my plants before planting, and I have utilized sex testing to good effect so I can maximize my limited garden growing space. If you have enough room to grow your plants and would like to keep costs to a minimum, you can sex your plants later on by using visual inspection (see page 95).

Protect and Transplant

It's now time to plant your cannabis toddlers in their final home. And for those of you planting clones—this is where you start. Purchase your clones close to when you intend to plant out in the garden. If your outdoor planting time window is more than five days out, you should plant your clones in a quart-size plastic or paper planter with high-quality planting mix to keep your plants happy and growing while they wait to be placed in their permanent garden home. Once all danger of frost is past, the soil is about 70°F, and daylight is more than twelve hours per day, it's planting time. Since you've carefully selected the spot for your cannabis and have amended the soil, all the hard work has been done. By now your cannabis plant should have at least two sets of true leaves, a well-established root mass, and be at least 6 inches tall, likely even taller.

Harden Them Off

If you've been nurturing your cannabis youngsters inside, it's important to harden them off prior to planting outside in their final home. *Hardening off* is a common garden term that refers to the act of moving plants outdoors for specific lengths of time, so they can become acclimatized to sunlight, temperature, and cooler nights. Since plants are at the mercy of their environment, they need time to adjust to sudden changes in their surroundings to avoid a setback in their health. Indoor temperatures are usually pretty consistent, while outdoor temperatures will likely have larger swings, especially in spring. Sunlight is much stronger light than most artificial lighting,

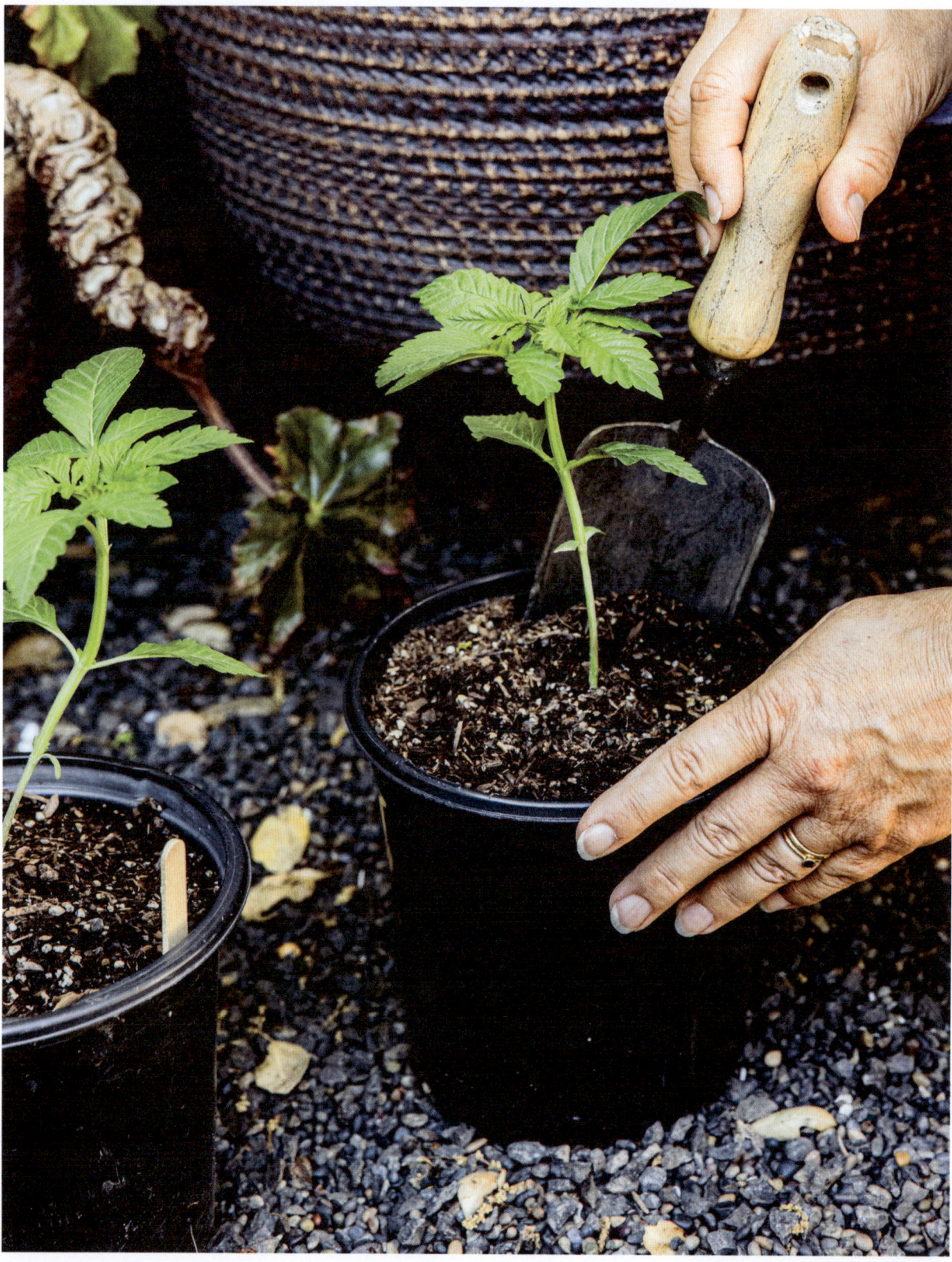

so hardening off your clones and seedlings will transition them to the stronger light of the sun. Hardening off is as important for clones as it is for seedlings to avoid transplant shock.

Help your indoor babies adjust to the outside conditions by giving them a couple of days while still in their pots in the place in which they will be growing after they are planted. If the weather is mild and consistent, leave them out for a day or two. If the weather is stormy or suddenly dips in temperature, bring the babies back inside during the bad weather spell, then set them out again the next day. Once the little plants have had time to get accustomed to the outside weather, you can plant them into their final homes. For those of you planting directly in the ground, it's wise to gauge the soil temperature before planting your seedlings. Stick your fingers into the soil a couple inches down from the surface. No need for a thermometer—just approximate the temperature with your hand. Is it cool? Warm? Lukewarm? This is great. Is it cold—less than 60°F? If so, allow the soil to warm up before planting your cannabis plant. If you love technology or just want extra assurance that the soil is an appropriate temperature for planting, you may use a soil thermometer to measure the soil temperature. If you suspect that you will have cold soil when it's time to plant, you can help warm the soil by laying out a black plastic sheet on the soil surface to speed up the soil temperature rise. Check the soil temperature again after several days, removing the plastic when the soil has warmed to 70°F at the surface.

It's Time to Dig

Planting the cannabis is easy and affords you the chance to inspect and admire your plants up close before they get tucked into their new earthy homes. If you're a curious person like me, you'll naturally take a look at those beautiful roots, being careful, of course, not to disturb the taproot. Those roots will be white and branched, and should be holding the soil mass together. You may notice some fuzzy white growth on the top or sides of the soil ball; this is very likely the mycorrhizae (the growing body of beneficial soil fungus) that is routinely added to planting mixes designed for cannabis. No need to worry—this is a good thing for your weed baby. Those beneficial fungus threads are in a friendly win-win relationship with your cannabis plant and will help your weed thrive in the garden.

Dig an appropriate-size hole for your little plant, aiming for twice as wide and as deep as the root-ball. Carefully remove your cannabis

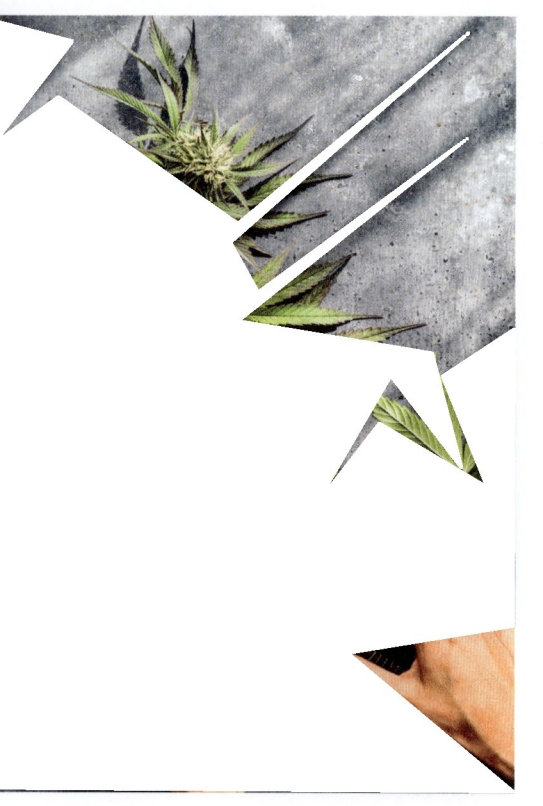

plant from its quart-size pot, keeping the root-ball intact, and place the plant in the center of the hole. Make sure the shoulder of the root-ball soil block is at the same level as the surrounding soil. Gently press the soil around your plant's soil block, then thoroughly but gently water the new plant to settle the soil and remove any larger air holes between the native soil and the root-ball. Keep your cannabis plant evenly moist, watering gently but frequently for the first several weeks if you don't have rainfall. After a brief period of settling in, your cannabis plant will send its roots out and begin to put out new green growth at a rapid pace. Remember that your plant will be 6 to 13 (or more) feet tall in a few months, so strap in for some Jack-and-the-Beanstalk–level growth.

Keep a Photo Record

I encourage you to take photos of your plants every couple of days or at least once a week. Not only will you have something amazing to show your canna-curious friends (yeah . . . I grew that!), but it will serve you well in improving your grow for next year by documenting your steps. Take time to admire your plants. Not only with this keep you in touch with what your plants need, you'll have fun, too. I think these plants are irresistibly pretty.

GROWING UP   For the first several weeks in their new homes, your cannabis plants will be establishing their root mass and growing quickly. Think of them as happy, healthy first graders going off to school. During this early growth stage, concentrate on creating a consistent environment. Cannabis is a vigorous grower, with robust resilience to many different conditions—no coddling needed. That said, it's important to pay attention to your young plants and give them the support they need for the best start in the garden. Keep your plants evenly watered but never soggy. Cannabis requires consistent moisture throughout its life—especially so during the fast growth of juvenility. If your little plant experiences moderate winds, they will be just fine. However, if the weather takes a turn for the worse with stormy weather—strong winds, hail, or heavy rains—it would be wise to protect your plants with an overturned bucket or a supported tarp to help prevent damage. And as soon as the storm subsides, remove any coverings.

Leaves and More Leaves

Young cannabis leaves are gloriously green and fresh. Clones will come with mature leaves already present on the little plants, while seedlings will have seed leaves in addition to true leaves. Cannabis leaves are veined, lightly textured palmate leaves with serrate edges. The maximum number of lobes on any one plant is nearly always between five and thirteen and is predetermined by the cannabis strain's genetics.

Your plant will move through the early juvenile growth stage quickly, and each successive generation of leaves will emerge bigger and more lobed until they reach the fan leaf stage. A full-grown fan leaf can be quite large—bigger than an adult hand with fingers outstretched. These are the famous, easily recognizable leaves that we associate with this plant. Pay attention to the lush green fan leaves in the vegetative stage. Cannabis leaves are important indicators of health for your plants and will communicate clearly how your plant is doing and what it might need help with. There are rarely many problems in the early veg stage—we'll explore more about addressing problems in the next chapter. Even though the easygoing early veg stage is usually vigorous and happy for your plants, it pays to be observant. As a gardener, your role is to pay attention to your plants and give them support when they need it. Plants, not the gardener, do the work. Get to know your cannabis plant leaves and you will be a more effective gardener.

Nurturing young cannabis plants offers serendipitous benefits to the home cannabis gardener. You'll quickly realize the fecundity of your plant when every day brings a new burst of green leaves. Pick a few healthy leaves for a refreshing, soothing herbal tisane (see page 175). Throw some fresh, young leaves in the blender with frozen fruit for a smoothie. Hone your floral arranging skills using cuttings from your plant. Even placing one perfect fan leaf in a little vase is a feast for the eyes.

Pinch It Back

Your plant will gain both height and width during the veg stage, branching out to become a multiple-stemmed herbaceous shrub. After a month or so in the ground, you will need to decide whether to pinch back your plant; this simply means removing a small section of the tallest, topmost growing tip of a plant in order to shape its growth. While this topic is relevant to both seed- and clone-grown cannabis, it's perhaps a bit more important for seed-grown cannabis, since these plants tend to grow tall and large. Before you get too worried about this subject, take heart that there is no absolute decision to be made. You can have perfectly good cannabis from a pinched back or naturally growing plant, in spite of the big deal that many commercial growers make about this subject. You're a gardener, not a farmer, so relax and focus on enjoying your plants.

Most types of cannabis will grow into a classic pyramidal Christmas tree shape if left alone. The exception to this is the sativa-dominant plants that are more naturally multiple branched. The natural growth pattern for most hybrid cannabis has a straight up-and-down central stalk with lateral branches. The plant is skinniest at the top with gradually larger width as your eye moves down to the ground. This is an efficient design, from the plant's perspective, since it allows maximum light to shine on each part of the plant. Imagine looking down at a mature plant, with your eyes dead center. You'll see a circle of green, with each leaf jockeying into position to get light. Each branch tip is the growth edge for that branch, and the biggest growth edge of all is at the very top of the plant. The plant is managing its growth by sending certain chemicals (auxins) to the part of the plant that is farthest away from the root, using gravity as stimulus. As the cannabis plant matures and flowers, this topmost branch, the apical tip, will also produce the biggest set of flowers—called the apical cola. (We'll explore more about flowering in the next chapter; I mention it here only to set the stage for our understanding of pinching back.)

Pinching back a young plant removes the plant's growth tip. Cannabis responds to this stimulus by growing two new, smaller, lead growth tips. Where there was one lead, there will now be two coequal leads. This is called topping the cannabis plant, because you are removing the top of the plant. There are reasons why some growers prefer to trim their cannabis plants in this way, while others choose not to. When you pinch back a cannabis plant, causing two leads to grow rather than one, the overall shape of the plant gets bushier and somewhat shorter. This results in slightly smaller but more numerous flower clusters at the end of the growing season. This can be a helpful practice if you live in an area in which you expect cool or moist conditions during harvest because smaller colas are less prone to mold problems than fatter colas. Pinching off can also be a helpful practice if you want to have a wider, bushier, shorter plant at maturity. The resulting smaller, more numerous colas resulting from pinching off are either a blessing or a curse, depending on what you are going for. If you want to have that big, fat, photo-worthy apical cola, then by all means—let your plant do what it does naturally and grow a huge apical cola.

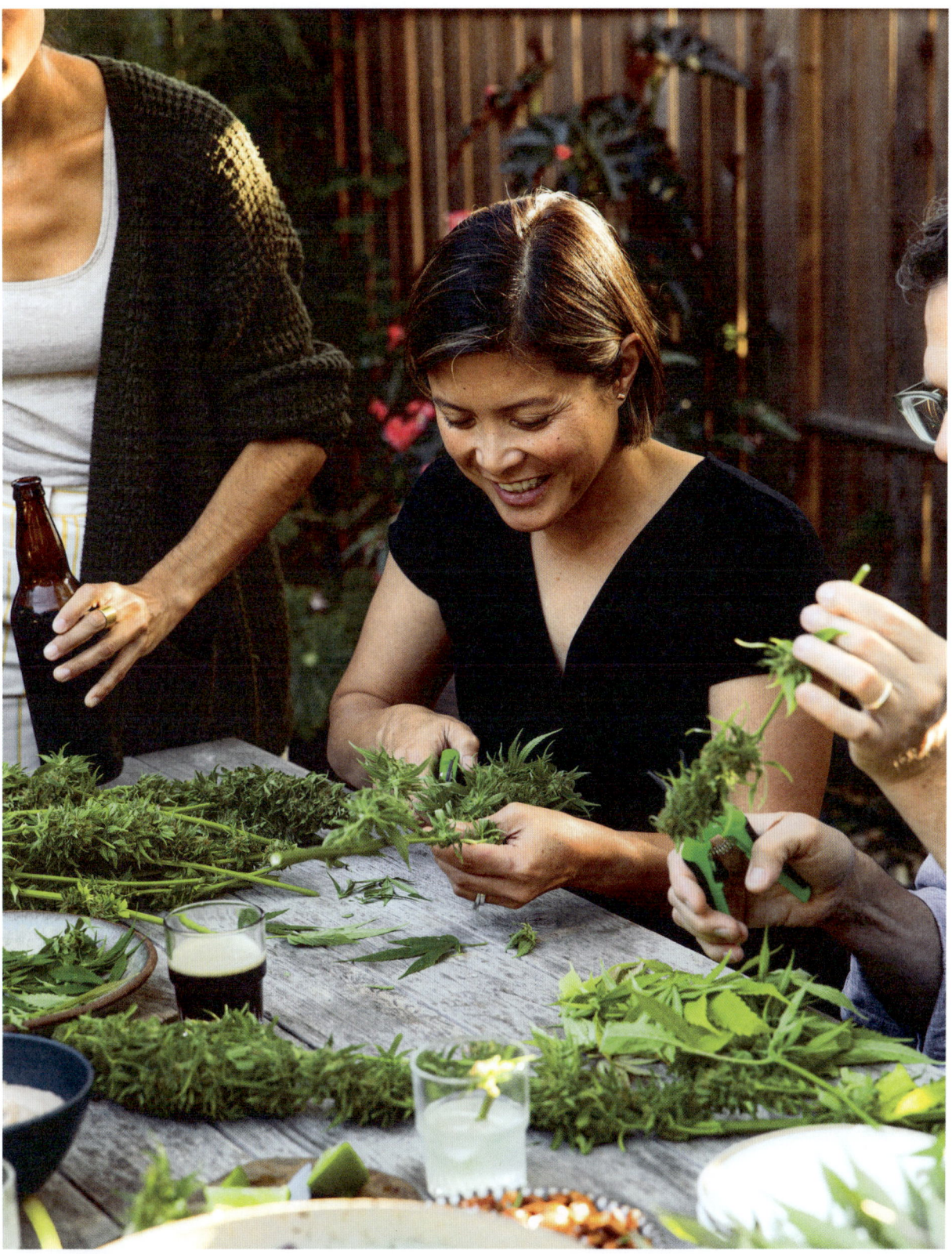

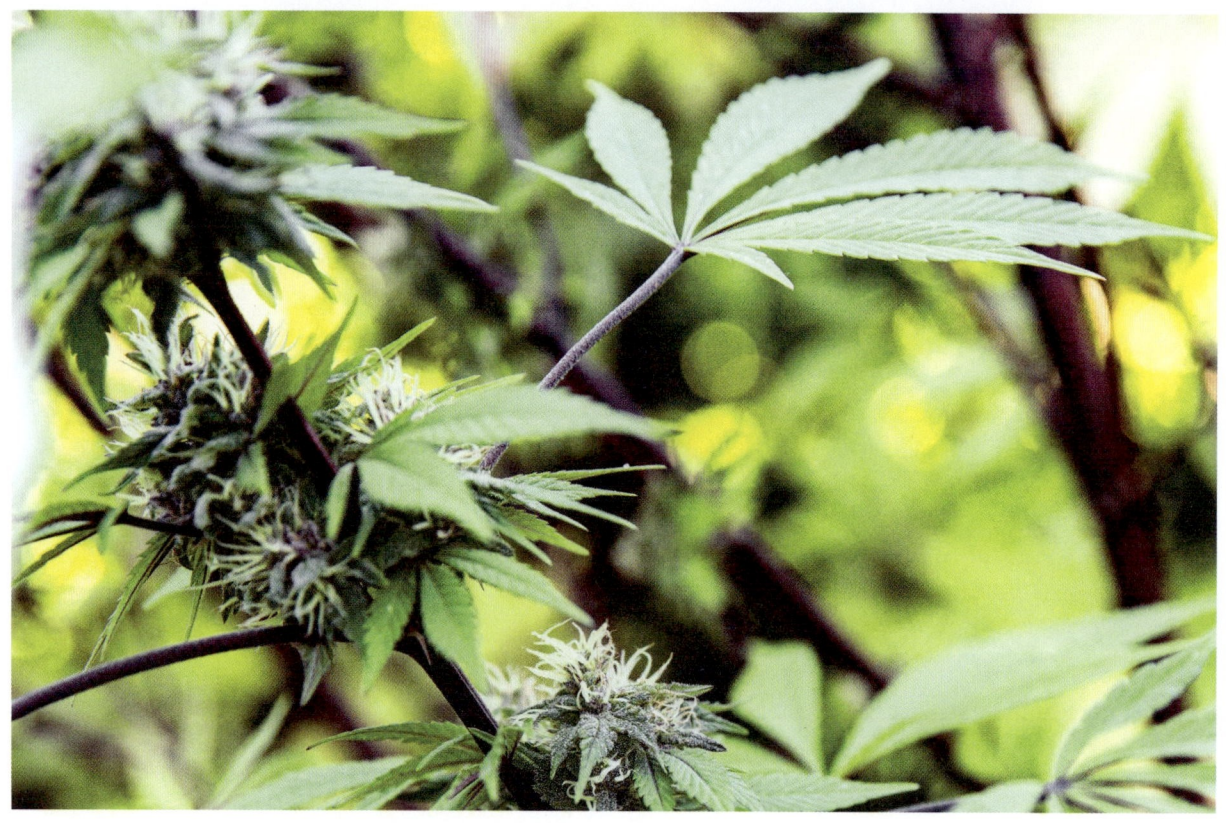

Another consideration is whether to aim for a more weather-resistant, mature plant. Strong winds are unkind to bushy cannabis plants with a lot of heavy buds, although proper staking will offset this risk. A mature pyramid-shaped cannabis plant will resist damage better than a bushy, fat plant. Most sources agree that both pinched and unpinched outdoor-grown cannabis will bear similar bud yields, all other conditions being equal.

The technique of pinching back is super simple—but it needs to happen at the right time in a plant's life. Pinch back after your plant is well established in its final growing spot—but before it is more than 3 or so feet tall and certainly well before any flowers begin to form. A good rule of thumb is to wait until the plant has between three and five nodes, the spots on the stem where leaves emerge. Remove the very tip of the plant, either with your finger and thumbnail or with clean pruning shears. You need to remove only the top inch or less of the plant to disrupt the lead and cause a bifurcation in the stem, the spot where two new lead branches will emerge. Be sure to observe the spot you intend to cut—it should be just ahead of where a new set of leaves will emerge from the plant. You may repeat this technique on a few other larger branch tips for an even bushier plant. Don't overthink it. You can't mess this up too much. This technique may sound familiar to more experienced gardeners, since this is the exact same technique used in producing bushier mums, begonias, basil, petunias, zinnias, cosmos, impatiens, and dahlias, to name a few. If you have the space to grow more than one plant, I suggest you try both techniques. Pinch one plant back and leave the other to grow naturally. Maybe you'll have better results with one style or the other. Remember—there is no such thing as perfect here. Either way can work—and with each season of gardening, you'll gain insight into what works best for you and your garden.

Raise Them Up

While your young cannabis plants are growing tall, they don't need staking. A naturally shrubby cultivar may not need staking either. Clones are often shrubbier and denser growing than seedlings, so take this into consideration as well. Is your plant in an area that is protected from wind? This is another reason to be more casual with staking.

However, it is important to peer into the future and consider how best to support your plants when they will be fully loaded with heavy blossoms. There is no perfect staking method—lots of different things can work. Let's explore a couple of practical options for supporting your plants as they mature.

Bamboo pole. Your cannabis plant—especially a naturally growing, unpinched plant—will have a strong, somewhat flexible central stem. A sturdy, smooth 6- to 8-foot bamboo pole makes an excellent support. Place the pole a couple of inches out from the central stem and secure it into the surrounding soil until it feels stable and firm. Use soft twine or gardener's tape to loosely tie your cannabis stem to the pole. Remember that your little plant's central stem will widen and stiffen during its life, so do not use a rigid or inflexible product to tie your plant to the stake. This pole will be enough of a support for most of your plant's life. Additional small stakes can be added at the periphery of the plant as its flowers mature and grow heavy.

Tomato cage. A large tomato cage is a great support for weed plants. There are a number of large-format, sturdy cages from which to choose. Look for cages with large openings, smooth surfaces, and a height of at least 4 feet—the bigger the better. The goal is to offer support for the heavily laden flowering branches, and a wide, strong tomato cage is a good option. When the plant is still small, set the cage around the central stem. Gently guide any little branches through the openings of the cage.

Wire fencing. Sturdy metal fencing material is widely available at hardware stores, home improvement stores, and feed stores. This stiff fencing that has large (6-inch or more) square openings is often sold in large rolls or in precut panels. Place a 3- to 4-foot circle around each young plant and secure the cut ends of the fencing together to create an enclosure. Gently guide young branches through the squares. This will allow the plant lots of room to grow up and out, offering support throughout the life of your lovely lady.

Metal, wood, or PVC structure. If you have the time or inclination, try your hand at building a structure to support your plant. As long as your structure is freestanding and offers support to your plant, the sky's the limit. And if you have a generous gardening budget, consider investing in a garden obelisk. There are also a number of stylish wrought iron options available. Grow your weed with beauty in mind.

Feed the Soil

If you used fresh, quality planting mix or nicely amended your garden soil with compost, you will not need to do any fertilizing during the veg stage. Let your eyes be your guide to what your plant needs. Your lady's leaves will tell you everything you need to know—if you pay attention. If you rushed the soil prep stage and didn't amend your soil with compost before planting, you can always top-dress with compost now to give your plants a boost. The juvenile stage is when your fast-growing plants will need lots of nitrogen, and compost is a fabulous natural source of nitrogen. I avoid mineral or chemical fertilizers altogether, preferring to feed my plants with compost. A foliar feed (spraying leaves with a solution) from compost tea can be a wonderful probiotic health aid for your plants, giving them a quick boost of helpful microbes. (See chapter 5 for more specific instructions on compost teas and foliar feeding.)

The Right Way to Water

Keeping your cannabis plants evenly moist is key to their health. Those of us living in wet summer areas may be able to rely on rainfall alone to sustain the lush growth of our plants. For those in dry summer regions, setting up a good watering system is important. I have a small garden and enjoy daily visits to my plants. Watering by hand gives me time to pay attention to the plants, noticing any little issues and dealing with them before they turn into problems. If you see yellowing leaves in the juvenile growth stage, the most likely culprit is overwatering. If you see wilting leaves, make sure that you are keeping the plant's soil evenly moist but never soggy. When you water, take care to avoid soaking the leaves of the plant. Keep the ground moist and the leaves dry for best mold resistance.

Just in Case

Alas, sometimes a plant dies despite the best efforts of a gardener. Maybe there was a freak hailstorm and your weed got pummeled. Maybe your dog got a little too excited about digging in the freshly amended soil, and your cannabis plant got ejected from its earthen home. No matter the reason, you can recover if it's early enough in the season. July 1 is the cut-off date for planting outdoors in the Northern Hemisphere (January 1 for the Southern Hemisphere). If you live in a mild winter area, your growing season is long enough to replant with a regular cannabis clone or seedling. If you live in a cold winter region or it's later than July 1, consider planting an auto-flower. Auto-flowers finish quickly, so you can get a harvest before the growing season ends.

GROWER INSIGHTS
Drew Farwell

Drew Farwell spent his childhood in Maryland, his teen years in Washington state, then attended the University of Hawaii. He fell in love with surfing and the Hawaiian outdoors and has been in Oahu ever since. He began growing his own weed several years ago. He is enthusiastic about growing unique local cultivars acquired from the Oahu cannabis community. His greatest joy as a home grower is that cannabis is easy to grow, because Hawaii's climate offers the sun, water, and warmth that cannabis needs. Hawaii has two cannabis growing seasons—the long season (late March to October) and the short season (November through February). For the long season he loves Thai Stick and any other sativa-dominant strain. For the short season he has been growing indica-dominant strains and auto-flowers. Auto-flowers in particular do well in the short season as they will flower and finish well with Hawaii's small seasonal light fluctuations.

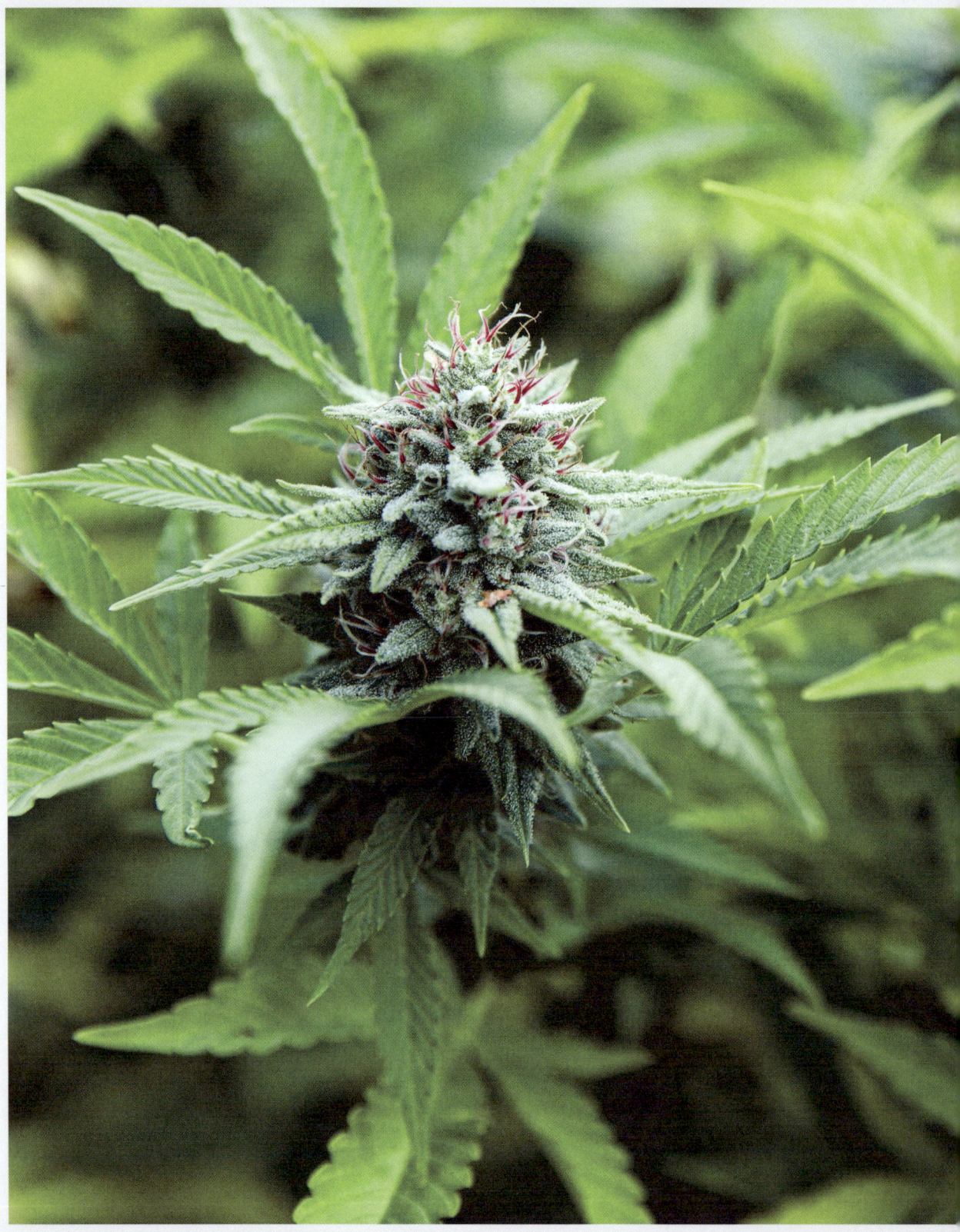

CHAPTER 5

The Flowering Stage:

From Blossom to Bud

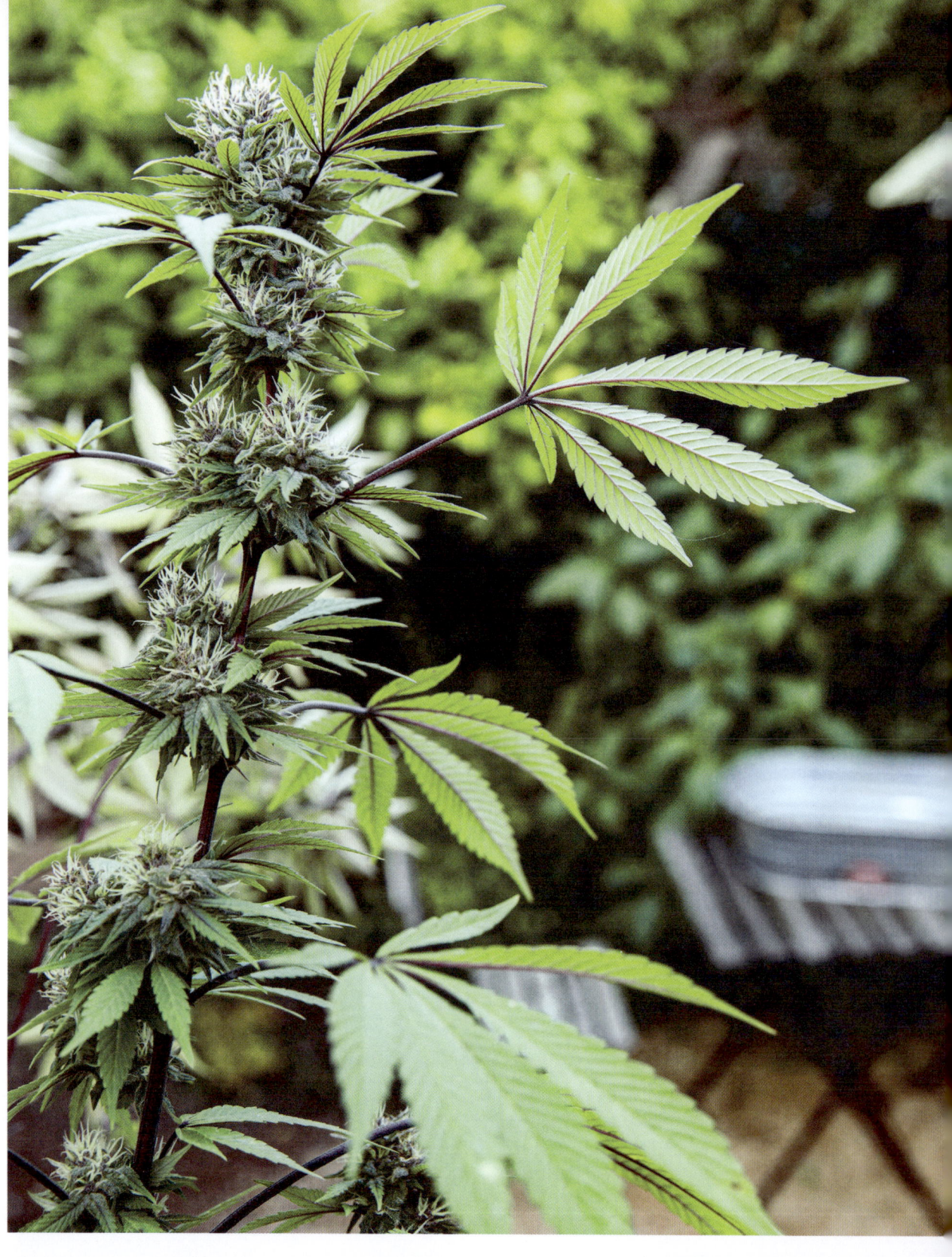

It's summer, and your cannababies are growing up. You've offered your little seedlings the best care—rich, well-draining soil; plenty of sun and fresh air; the gentle support of a strategically placed stake; and consistent water. The summer sun has been gracing your plants with plenty of light energy, and they have responded with lush green leaves, a stout central stalk, strong branches, and radiant beauty. Welcome to the flowering stage!

FROM TEEN TO OLD AGE

Your plants are all grown up now—they are likely bigger than you. If you've been enjoying frequent forays into your garden, there will come a day when you walk out to greet your plants, and something looks a little different. You will notice that the ends of the branches seem to be thickening up, looking a little fuzzy at the tips. You'll see that the newest leaves emerging from the ends of the branches are not as huge as the rest of the fan leaves. Something just seems a little different—poised for a change. Your ladies are teenagers now, so get ready for some drama! There are lots of exciting moments in the teen years, for both cannabis and people alike. Pay attention to your maturing plants during the flowering stage to stay ahead of common problems that can arise as your lovely ladies pour their energy into flower production and anticipate the end of their natural lives. In this chapter, we will learn about the second half of your weed's life as the plants bloom, set seed, and die. By continuing your good natural gardening practices, you will help guide your weed plants through healthy adulthood and into a rich harvest.

Let the Flowering Begin

When can you expect your plants to start flowering? That depends primarily on where you live, especially regarding your latitude. There is one thing that triggers blooming: darkness. In nature, cannabis originated in an area with distinct seasonal variations. The change in light from high summer to fall, with its shorter days and longer nights, is what signals the cannabis plant to bloom, get fertilized, and set seed: winter is coming. As explained earlier, cannabis is a photoperiod plant, responding to the seasonal triggers of increasing darkness to begin blooming. While many say that changes in the quality of the daylight trigger cannabis to bloom, it is more rightly understood as increasing periods of uninterrupted darkness. When there are more than twelve hours of uninterrupted darkness per night, your weed will start blooming. The exception is auto-flowering cannabis, which is not triggered to bloom by seasonal light changes (see page 71).

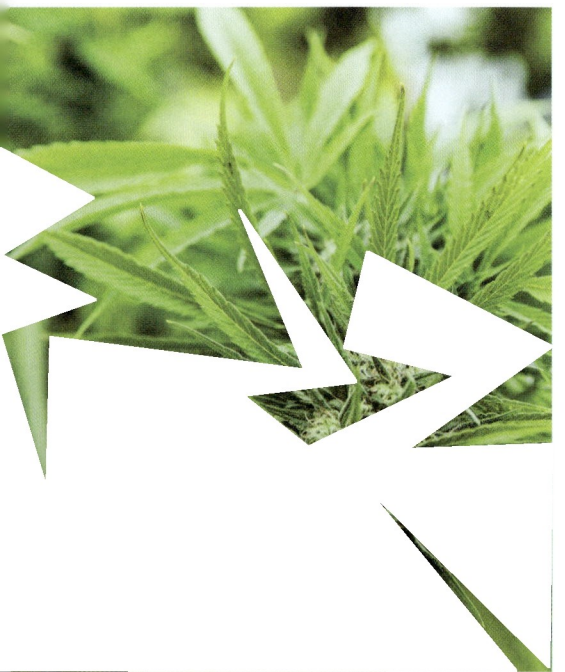

The latitude you inhabit has an impact on the date your cannabis will bloom because of the differences between regions in day and night length. If you have connections to growers in different parts of the world, you'll notice that those in lower latitudes will be done harvesting their sparkly weed earlier than those farther away from the equator. Although I discuss how to harvest cannabis in greater depth in chapter 7, I will offer a quick word here on how long you can expect it to be until you pick your bud. The length of time for your flowers to reach maturity is largely dependent on the plant's genetics. In general, cultivars with genetics from sunny, warm climates will take longer to mature, while cultivars hailing from cooler climates with shorter summers will finish more quickly. As a ballpark measure, cannabis will finish flowering from September 15 to November 1 in the Northern Hemisphere and from March 15 to May 1 in the Southern Hemisphere.

I want to offer you encouragement: just relax and focus on your plants. If you observe them daily, you'll become aware of the important growth stages. As a cannabis gardener, you get to hang out with these beautiful plants and learn from them. That is one of the joys of being an outdoor cannabis gardener—nature takes care of so many of the details. Your job is to keep your ladies happy and unpollinated until their blossoms are richly fragranced and sparkly with trichomes.

Changes to the Leaves

A remarkable transformation takes place during the beginning of flowering. The vigorous growth of the plant slows as the plant moves into the final stage of its life. Once the plant switches into flowering mode, the plant is in a death spiral—and this is a good thing. Remember, cannabis is an annual plant; it's designed to sprout, grow, mature, and die in under a year. Let's explore how you can expect your plant to change in the flowering stage.

You'll notice that the new leaves unfurling on the ends of the branches grow more densely. As flowering proceeds, the leaves will emerge smaller and smaller still, until the sugar leaves emerge—the smallest leaves of all. Sugar leaves are petite, have fewer lobes than the mature fan leaves, and are clustered under and in the flowers. They are called sugar leaves because they look as if they are covered with sugar—all sparkly and glistening white in the sun. But what looks like glittering sugar is actually a thick coating of structures called trichomes (page 120). These are tiny little structures that cover the upper surface of sugar leaves and flower parts. Trichomes are filled with the resins containing the cannabinoids and terpenes that weed is so famous for. Your plants will continue to grow during the flowering stage, but at a slower pace than in the frantic, fast growth of the vegetative stage.

Male or Female: How to Tell the Sex

In the flowering stage, flower clusters emerge in clumps at the ends of the branches. Each female flower has two fluffy, pale stigmas emerging from the bract-covered ovule—this is where a seed would form if the flower were pollinated. Each flower is rather small—¼ to ½ high at maturity—but grows in tight clusters of buds to form impressive inflorescences (complete flower clusters) called colas, which are usually found at the end of a branch. Colas are why we grow cannabis.

At the beginning of the flowering stage, the female flowers emerge as fuzzy little pom-poms at the branch tips. The fuzzy part is the mass of stigmas emerging from the ovules. Stigmas and ovules are parts of the female cannabis flowers. Most cannabis cultivars have white stigmas, but some varieties have pink, orange, or lavender stigmas. As the colas mature, you will notice they are growing longer and denser, are packed with buds, and have the beginnings of sparkle when they are in full sun. They're getting fragrant, too, especially in the heat of the day. If you planted regular (non-feminized) seed and did not do genetic sex testing early on, you will need to be on the lookout for males.

Male and female cannabis plants will look much the same in their youth. But as they enter the late veg stage, a few differences emerge. Look for preflowers—they are little flowers that emerge from the crotch between the main stem and a leaf node, near the top of the plant. If they have fuzzy stigmas emerging from their tips, they're female, but if they remain ball shaped, they are males (see www.pennybarthel.com for an image of a male flower). Cannabis is a wind-pollinated plant. As such, male cannabis plants make sure that their pollen has the best chance of finding a lovely lady to pollinate. They do this by growing taller and skinnier than the same-cultivar females, and they flower earlier and longer than the females. If one of your canna-teens seems extra tall, pay attention to the emerging flowers. Male flowers form first on the top part of the main stem, with the flowers forming not on branch tips but clustered loosely around the main stem. The immature male buds look like tiny balls on slim stems, turning upward, unfurling five slim petals around the stamens. Then they release pollen to the wind. If you find a male plant in your garden, don't allow it to bloom, unless you want seeds from your female plants. Boy, bye! Yank that male plant up by the roots and use any leaves that have some sparkly trichomes to make Cannabutter (page 160) or Cannabis Concentrate (page 156) for salves.

Cannabis Seeds for Next Season

If you are an adventurous cannabis gardener and would like to produce your own seed, you can! Grow a male cannabis plant in isolation, making sure that you have contained its pollen so that you don't inadvertently pollinate your neighbor's grow. Consider growing your male plant in a hoop tent with fabric that will keep the pollen inside. When your male plant's flowers open, gather some of the powdery pollen onto a fine paint brush and carefully apply it to one section of flowers on a branch of your female plant. Tie a bit of twine to the pollinated branch so you know where to look for seeds during harvest. The rest of the female's flowers will remain unpollinated and product good-quality bud. Collect and save any resulting seeds in a dry, cool, dark spot for planting next season.

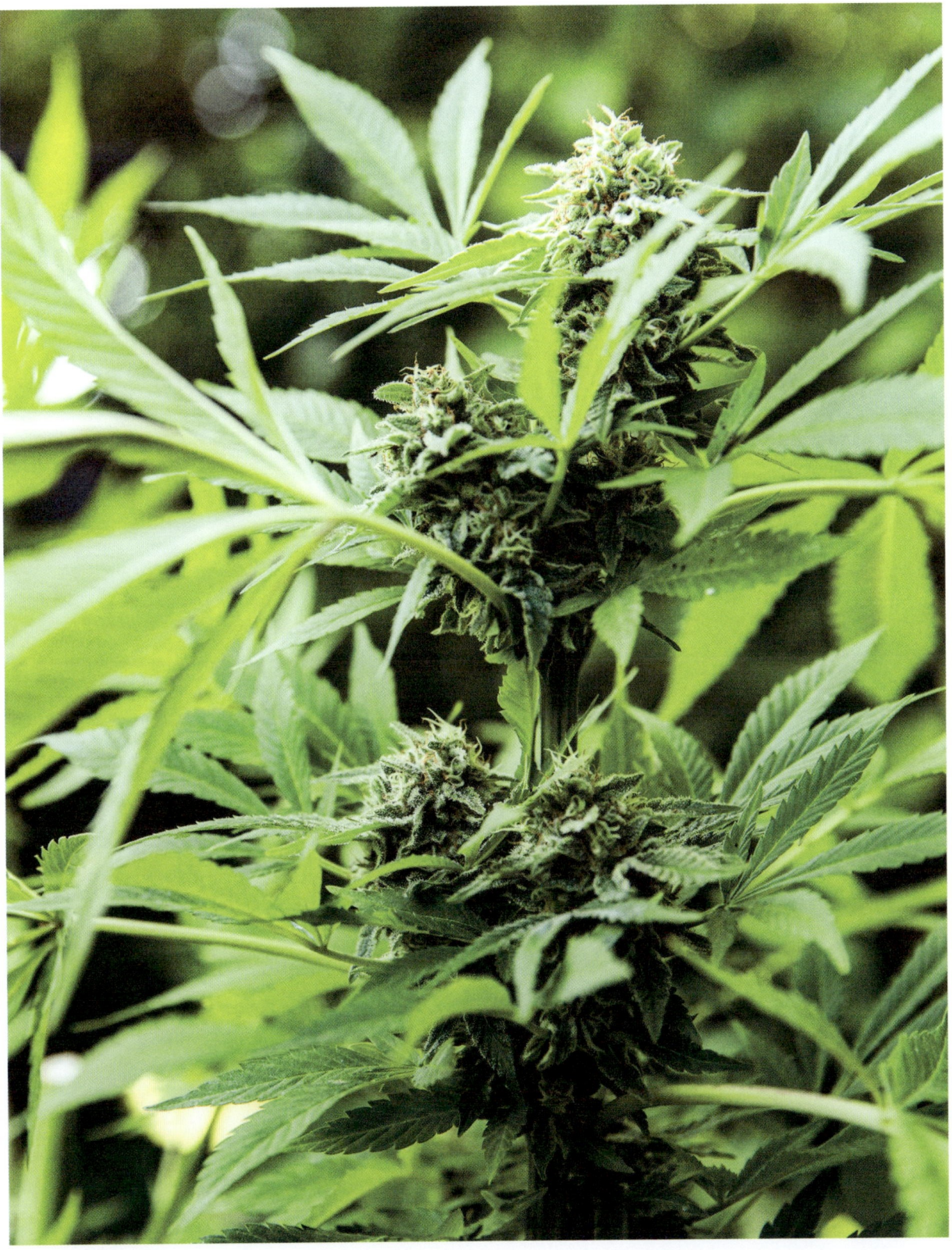

THE IMPORTANCE OF WATERING

As summer heat reaches peak temperatures, it is important to keep your plants happy—and proper watering is a vital component of caring for your grown-up ladies. Cannabis is a resilient plant and can withstand significant heat and drought, but temperatures over 85°F can cause your plant to need extra moisture. If you notice your cannabis plants wilting, this is a sign of dehydration and should be avoided, but your plants should spring back to good health quickly after being watered. One of the best parts of properly prepared soil is that it acts like a natural sponge. Good humus-rich soil will effectively soak up and hold water without being soggy. Summer heat is where healthy seed-grown cannabis really shows off. That massive root-ball anchored by the soil-penetrating taproot is the best drought-insurance policy for your plants. Plants grown in containers will require more attentive watering, since the limited soil volume and variable temperatures in containers necessitate more water. Additionally, if your cannabis plant is growing in a felt planter or in an unglazed terracotta pot, water is likely to evaporate from the soil more quickly in hot weather. If you grow in a hot, dry summer area—places such as eastern Oregon and Washington, California's central valley, and much of Southern California—you will probably have to water consistently throughout the growing season. If you garden in a wet summer area, you will likely have to water your plants on an as-needed basis. Whatever your watering needs, there are some best practices for watering to keep your flowering cannabis healthy and happy in the heat.

As cannabis enters the flowering stage, its leaf structure becomes denser and more prone to trapping moisture. The flower buds forming on the ends of the branches can trap water and can be slow to dry out, especially as their colas swell to mature size. Watering the soil without constantly wetting the maturing plant is important during the flowering stage; your ladies need consistent moisture to keep actively growing, but keep the plant leaves and flower buds dry to prevent your aging plant from succumbing to fungal diseases. Cannabis plants in the flower stage are focusing their energy on blooming and maturing—leaving less of their energy available for the vigorous growth and disease resistance of the veg stage. Opportunistic fungal diseases thrive in moist conditions and can be a problem for aging cannabis plants, but good watering practices will help to prevent fungal attacks on your maturing ladies.

GIVE YOUR FLOWERING PLANTS A SNACK

Healthy soil will support your plants right through the flowering stage. There are a few boosts you can offer to your maturing cannabis teens to keep them in top shape. As I discussed in chapter 2, plants make their own food from sunshine, air, and water—any feeding you do to your plants is just providing several macro- and micronutrients. Healthy soils are complex, resilient ecosystems that work in real time to provide the nutrients that plants require, on demand. In the vegetative stage, the fast-growing plants need ample nitrogen along with all the other macro- and micronutrients in healthy soil. In the flowering stage, a plant's overall growth rate slows while it concentrates on creating flowers and all the fragrant resins that cover them. As a plant flowers, it will appreciate a little extra phosphorus and potassium in addition to modest amounts of nitrogen. Again, let me affirm that if you've been taking great care of your soil, you will not need to add anything to your flowering plant's soil—your rich, well-amended soil should feed your plants just fine. That said, cannabis plants have immune systems—just as we do—and as they age, they become more prone to disease. Sound familiar? We have more in common with plants than we realize. If you notice your plants looking a little lackluster or if you want to get ahead of any emerging disease states, I offer four suggestions: compost tea, top dressing, fish emulsion with kelp, and vermiculture (worm composting).

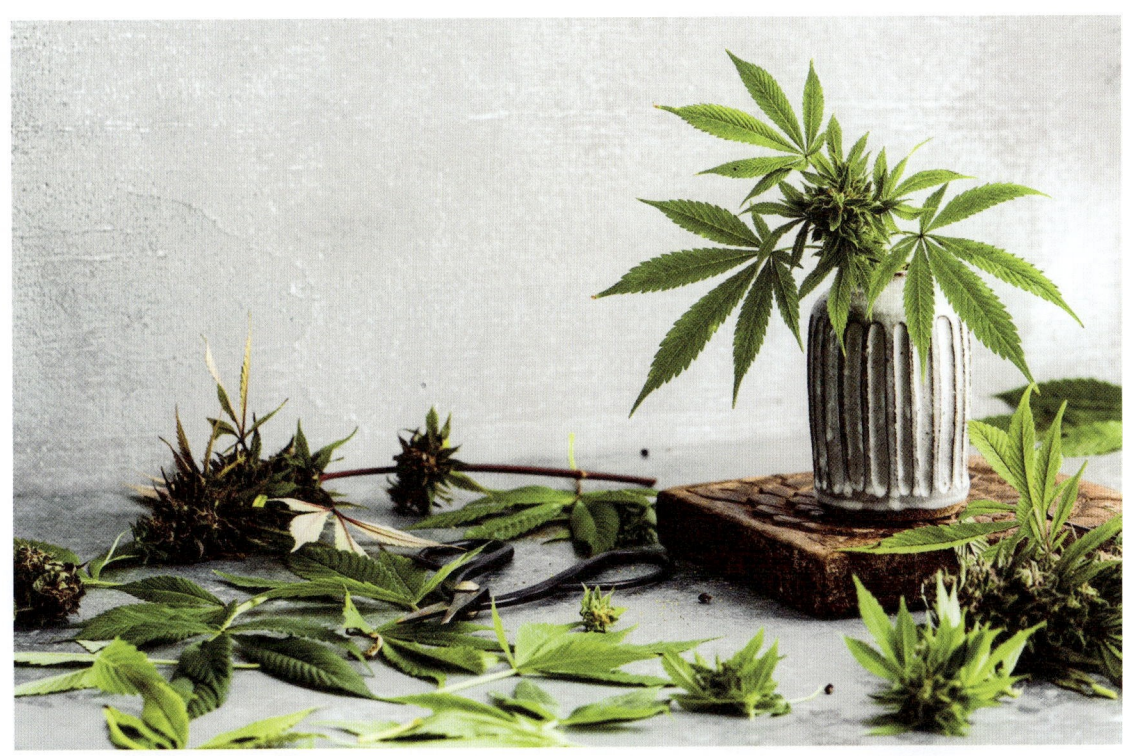

Brew Your Own Compost Tea (for your plants!)

Compost tea is exactly what it sounds like—you make a special "tea" out of compost and water. The key is to start with good-quality, living compost that is teeming with microscopic life. The naturally occurring microbial citizens of compost will vary, since each region's population of microbes is different. Your compost pile will differ from your neighbors', based on the different things that you each may have put into your piles. The exact type of life-forms in your compost doesn't matter terribly much, so no need to overthink it. Well-crafted compost tea will select for the bacteria that will aid your plant. The bacteria and other unseen organisms in the compost tea are allies for your plants and will offer them resistance to disease, especially fungal attacks. Compost tea kits are also available for purchase, making the set up a snap.

Here's how to brew your own compost tea:

SUPPLIES

Compost

Two 5-gallon buckets

Molasses or sugar

Aerator and pump

Mesh bag or cheesecloth

1. Start by adding a quart of high-quality living compost to a 5-gallon bucket.

2. Add non-chlorinated water to the compost in the bucket, leaving 3 to 4 inches of space at the top. If your source of water is chlorinated, as is the case with most municipal water, de-chlorinate it by filling a separate 5-gallon bucket with water and leave it exposed, outside for at least 24 hours prior to using it in your compost tea brew.

3. Stir in 2 tablespoons of molasses or sugar (this provides food for the microbes).

4. Place an aerator into the bucket and connect it to the pump to begin brewing. An aerator is an inexpensive device to keep air bubbles flowing through the solution.

5. Aerate the mixture, making sure it remains gently bubbling through-out the 24-hour incubation. The bubbles will keep the solution filled with air, bringing oxygen to the helpful microbes and allowing them to eat the sugars and multiply. Without the bubbles, the solution will quickly become anaerobic (oxygen poor). This will cause harmful bacteria to grow, making the tea smell really stinky, and become unhealthy for your plants.

6. Remove the aerator, strain the compost tea through a mesh bag or cheesecloth into a 5-gallon bucket, and it's ready to use. Use within a few hours for best results. Discard the solution if it smells stinky.

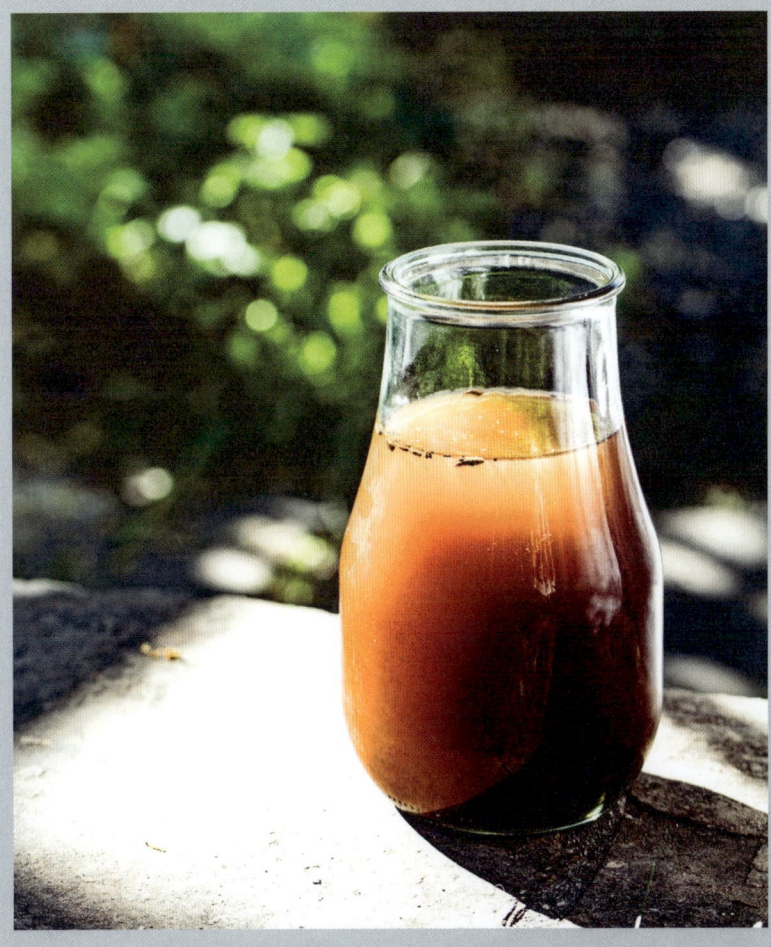

This finished compost tea will be filled with microbial life and nutrients for your plants. This is a potently alive solution, and the plants will love it. You can add this compost tea directly to the soil, adding a microbe boost to your soil ecosystem. When you add this to your plant's soil, it increases the overall fertility of the soil, making more mineral nutrients bioavailable to your plant.

If you want to give your plants a quick boost, try foliar feeding—spraying the compost tea directly on the leaves. The aging fan leaves will quickly respond to the foliar spray with renewed vigor and disease resistance. Strain some of the compost tea, put it into a fine rosette watering can or a pressurized spraying container, and wet your plants' leaves with the microbe-rich tea.

Boost with Top Dressing

You may feed your plants by top-dressing the soil around your cannabis plants. Top dressing is a common gardening technique for adding a boost of organic matter and fertility to the soil without digging it in. This is a great late-season trick, because it doesn't disrupt the roots while offering your hard-working soil microbes a midseason snack. Here's how to top-dress your plants: If you've mulched your plants (which I highly recommend; page 56), scrape away the mulch into a nearby mound. Sprinkle your compost around the root mass of the plant to the edges of the leaf line. Water in the compost, then restore the mulch that you'd previously scraped away. That's it—nature will do the work for you now.

Feed with Fish Emulsion

If your plants are showing signs of fatigue, you can also feed them a good-quality organic supplement, such as fish emulsion with kelp. Apply this supplement according to the directions on the label and use sparingly to be gentle on your soil's ecosystem.

Speed Things Up with Worms

Worm castings are hugely helpful to a soil's fertility. Worm castings are available for purchase at nurseries, or you can make your own with a worm compost system, also known as vermiculture. There are many DIY or commercially available vermiculture systems, mostly made up of two stacked, covered boxes, the top of which has drainage holes. Create a suitable home for your worms—usually red wrigglers—by combining shredded paper and kitchen scraps, then add the worms. Keep feeding the colony both dry and wet organics (no animal products though), and make sure the colony has lightly moist conditions but never gets too soggy. Keep it from overheating or freezing. What you're after is the dark, rich liquid that forms in the bottom bin. This is a terrific living tonic for your soil. You can also dilute the liquid castings in water and use the water as a foliar spray for your flowers and buds. Yes, you're spraying worm poop onto your plants, but that's okay. Worms have remarkable digestive systems; they excrete healthy, clean, biologically rich castings that will give your plants an immune boost.

SHAPE AND SUPPORT THEM

By the time your weed teens are flowering, they will have achieved their mature bush structure. Your ladies are all grown up and getting ready for the prom.

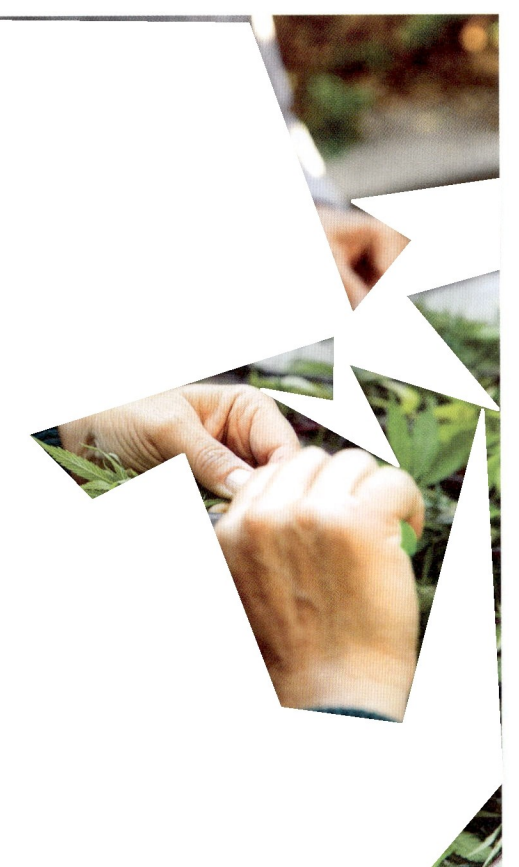

To Prune or Not to Prune

This is the ideal time to shape and support your cannabis to prepare for the last stages of flowering. Stand back and admire your weed plant—look at all those big fan leaves. They are the chief food factories for the plant, and they have been working hard all summer. The oldest fan leaves start to retire during this flowering period and may yellow. This is normal—and signifies that the plant is moving nitrogen from the oldest leaves into the newer fast-growing flower buds. There is no need to worry about a gradual lessening of the older leaves' vigor. Another reason the plant retires some of its leaves is that they are shaded out by new growth on the plant and so aren't able to earn their keep anymore. You may remove some of the fully shaded and yellowing fan leaves for best airflow—your plant can stand to lose some of its older fan leaves. I recommend that you ignore the advice of some growers who meticulously strip their plants of fan leaves. This is not how nature works—the healthy fan leaves are there for a reason and are needed for energy throughout the life of your plant.

If your plant is particularly dense and shrubby, consider removing some of the smaller branches that are fully shaded by other more vigorous branches. This will encourage more resources to go into the healthy maturation of the bigger, sun-blessed colas. It will also bring much-needed airflow through the interior of the plant. Good airflow is the best way to stave off fungal attacks—a common problem in the flowering stage, especially in cool, wet conditions.

Raise Them Up

If you didn't set up a support system when you planted your seedling or clone, early in the flowering season is a great time to do some staking. If you provided supportive caging or staking early on, you may be all set for your plant's support needs. However, if you haven't staked your plant so far, take a moment to decide whether or not to provide more support to your lady. If you see big branches that look ready to grow dense, heavy colas, I recommend providing a stake for each large branch. If you pinched back the leading tip of your young plant, you'll likely have a rounded, top-heavy plant at maturity. These bushes do well with some support to the several lead branches.

One product is the Mighty Crop staking system. These are 12-inch-round, lightweight units that latch onto a stake and offer support to several branches. Three or four of these used with stakes would be an adequate, flexible support for your large outdoor plants. Whatever system you use to provide support to your plant, allow the branches to continue to sway in the breeze without rubbing against a rough surface—you want healthy, intact stalks to protect the plant from disease-introducing friction injuries.

DEALING WITH NUISANCES

Like all living things, cannabis plants have active immune systems. Healthy plants will fight off most pests on their own, especially if you've been giving them immune-boosting compost tea foliar sprays (see page 100). I am a huge believer in prevention, especially when it comes to plant health. Every time I tend to my soil, feeding it biologically rich compost, I prevent disease in my garden. I prefer to avoid pests and disease rather than treat for them. But even with the most careful and wholesome gardening, as your ladies age, they will become weaker and more prone to certain diseases. When this happens, plants will need a little extra care. A good resource for a more complete guide to pest management is the book *What's Wrong with My Marijuana Plant*.

Here are the most common issues you'll likely face with your cannabis plants and some natural treatment options.

Powdery Mildew

A common issue on cannabis is powdery mildew. Powdery mildew is a surface-growing fungal infection, caused by molds that are opportunistic pathogens, meaning that they are always around but only become a problem on susceptible leaves. Powdery mildew looks as if the sugar fairy had come out in the middle of the night and dusted the leaves with white powder. Powdery mildew grows when the leaf surface is consistently moist, and it is especially prevalent if the leaves are in the shade. Some plants, including sweet peas and squash, are especially vulnerable to powdery mildew, and cannabis can be as well. If you planted more than one strain, you may notice that one gets powdery mildew, while another one doesn't. Pay attention to which strains resisted better than others, taking notes for future growing seasons. Generally, dense, heavy colas and stout bushy plants are more prone to powdery mildew because they are more moisture trapping than the lankier, more loosely flowered plants. Certain climates—such as in the Bay Area and the coastal Pacific Northwest with their cool, foggy summers and cloudy winters—are more prone to powdery mildew outbreaks than dry, sunny climates. Growers in the muggy summers of the Northeast US also have problems with this disease. Powdery mildew likes leaf moisture, so poor airflow is a contributor to powdery mildew problems. It is not a systemic disease, though, and can be treated. Begin treating any outbreaks of powdery mildew by removing noticeably infected fan leaves. Spray the remaining affected leaves with a baking soda solution (1 teaspoon of baking soda dissolved in 1 gallon of water) once daily in the morning for three days, or until the powdery mildew fades. Baking soda is a mild base. When you spray it on your leaves, it changes the pH of your leaf surface and creates unfavorable conditions for the powdery mildew to grow. You may also use this spray as a preventive if you know that your area is prone to the disease. If you treat one plant for an active case of powdery mildew but your others don't yet show signs, consider offering them a preventive treatment. Biologically active foliar tea sprays offer natural resistance to powdery mildew (see page 100). Another treatment option is a neem oil spray, used per the manufacturer's instructions. Neem oil is a low-toxicity, natural product made from the oil of the neem tree. Neem oil spray can be a little smelly for an hour or two after application, but the odor fades pretty quickly.

Budworm

Another common problem for your flowering cannabis is the dreaded budworm. Not actually a worm, these little caterpillars are the larvae of several types of flying insects that develop in and eat the growing cluster of flower buds. They are annoying and leave behind little black pellets that stick to the resinous trichomes of your sugar leaves and buds. Not only are they a nuisance but they also offer a more serious problem: the injuries they cause to the cannabis tissues can introduce a systemic fungus that can rot your cannabis cola from the inside out. I know that there are budworms in my area, and I've experienced them on past cannabis grows. Because of this, I preventively treat my flower buds with a biological control. There is a particular species of bacteria, *Bacillis thuringiensis* (Bt), that can be prepared as a spray for your flower buds. This bacterium interacts with the larvae's digestion systems and causes the larvae to stop feeding and to die. Bt spray is best applied liberally to all the flower buds on a calm, windless morning. You will need to repeat applications of Bt once a week or so to effectively treat and prevent a budworm infestation. Because I took this preventive measure to ensure protection against budworms' damaging munching, I did not have any problems with this pest this past season. Neem oil spray is also an effective treatment for budworms and can be used in conjunction with Bt for an active infestation.

Bud Rot

Bud rot, or bot, is caused a number of pathogenic fungi, most notably *Botrytis cinerea*. Unlike powdery mildew, which is a surface-growing organism, bud rot is a systemic fungal infection, meaning that it gets into the whole plant's vascular system and grows throughout the plant. Bud rot is more likely to show up in larger, denser colas than in looser, fluffier colas (see photo at right). It is also more common in cannabis grown in cool, wet weather, in shady conditions, or in muggy, stifling weather. Good airflow helps keep bot in check, because excess moisture creates happy conditions for fungal growth. Infestation with budworm can also make bot more common because the injuries to the plant's tissues allow the fungus to gain entry to your plant's insides. By keeping your flower free of budworm, you will help prevent bud rot.

Remember to hang out with your ladies. They love your company. By observing their beautiful emerging flowers, you will be the first to notice bud rot. While you're looking at a cola, watch for little gray patches on your bud. Gently inspect the interior of the bud. Does the bud feel weak or look gray-beige rather than green? If so, you likely have the beginnings of bud rot. It's time to pinch out the infected spots. With your fingers, remove any infected bud tissue and discard it in the trash, not your compost. Because bud rot is a systemic issue, you can't directly treat the problem. If one blossom shows signs of bud rot, remove the infected part and watch and wait.

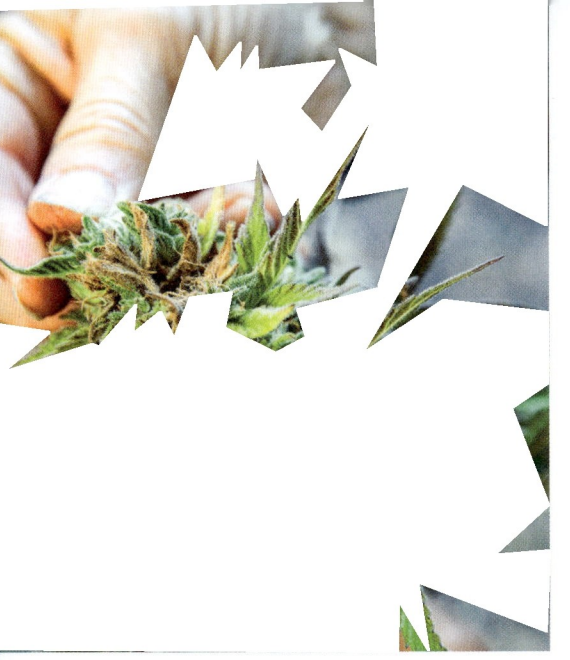

Keep water off your buds, improve airflow, and make sure your lady is in the clarifying sunshine. If you're gardening in a planter and you notice bud rot, try moving your lovely lady to a sunnier or breezy locale to finish flowering. And take note of which of your plants became infected and which ones didn't; some strains are more sensitive to bud rot than others. Keep track of which strains thrived in your area and compare notes with local outdoor growers to learn which ones work best in your local climate.

Mites

Cannabis growers in hot, dry areas have a greater likelihood of mite infestations. These tiny arachnids—spider relatives—are the sap-sucking denizens of the cannabis plant. There are different types of mites, but they all enjoy hot, dry conditions. Most healthy cannabis will keep mites in check, but these little creatures love a desert climate and can overwhelm some plants in hot, dry areas. Neem oil spray is a good treatment option to control a mite infestation.

Flying Insects

Some areas of the world with hot, humid summers may see a large swarm of insects from time to time. While well-attended cannabis is a vigorous grower and can outpace most pathogens, heavy insect populations may overwhelm your ladies. Cannabis can be grown under insect-control screening to prevent flying insects from overtaking your plants. Just be sure to allow your ladies to grow to full size with enough room under the protective fabric of an insect barrier. And, of course, make sure your screening allows airflow.

ENJOY YOUR BUDS

As late summer approaches, you will be nearing the twilight of the flowering period. Take time to enjoy your plants. If you can spare a couple of pretty branches, snip them and put them in a vase. They will be quite long-lasting, and they work well in combination with other late-summer flowers and greens. As a cannabis gardener, you have the special treat of harvesting some of your baby flower colas to use in tisanes (herbal teas). You can't buy fresh young cannabis bud; you need to grow your own. My outside-grown cannabis plants always have an abundance of flowers, and I like to harvest and freeze some for a tisane during the winter to remind me of the joys of summer (see page 172).

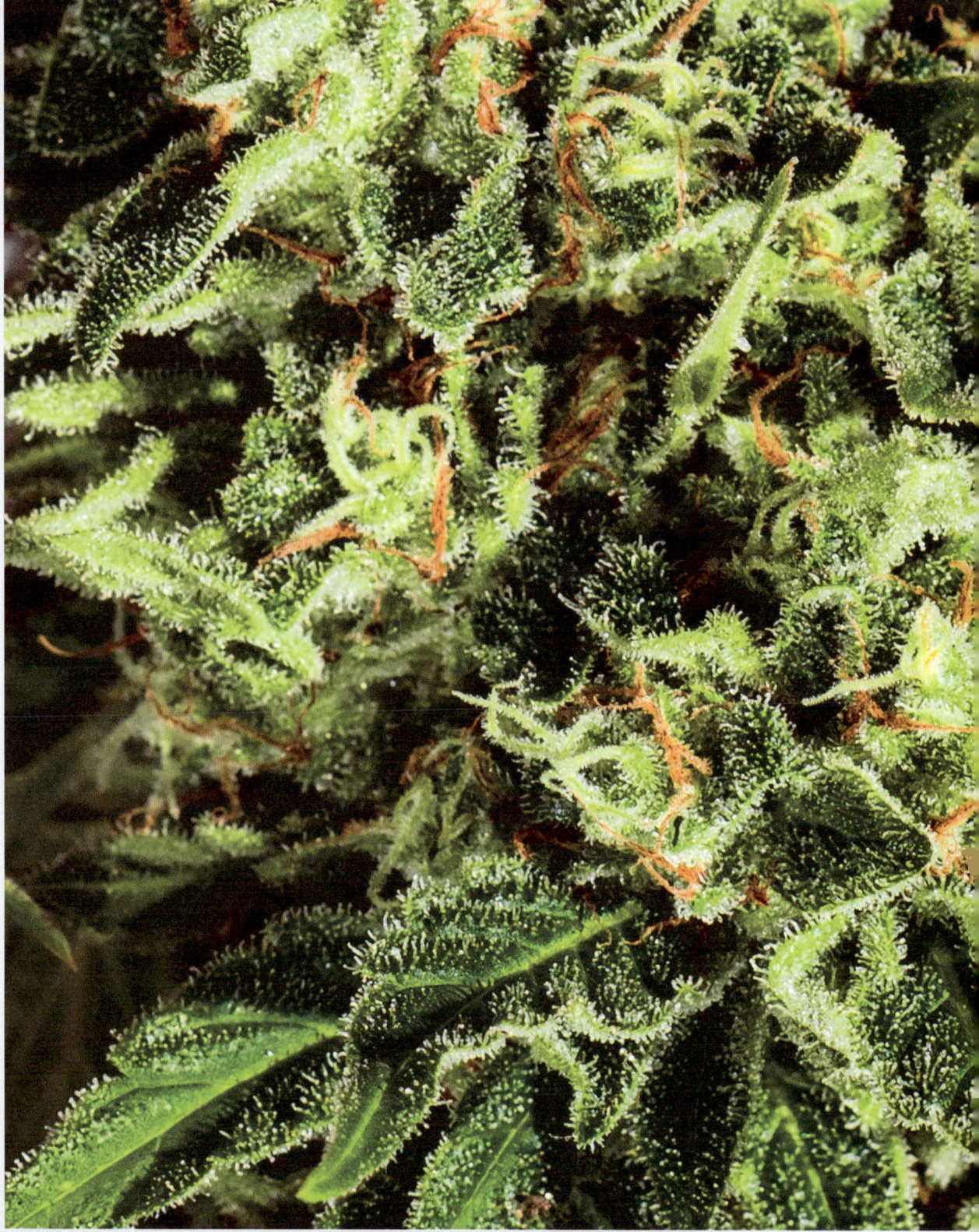

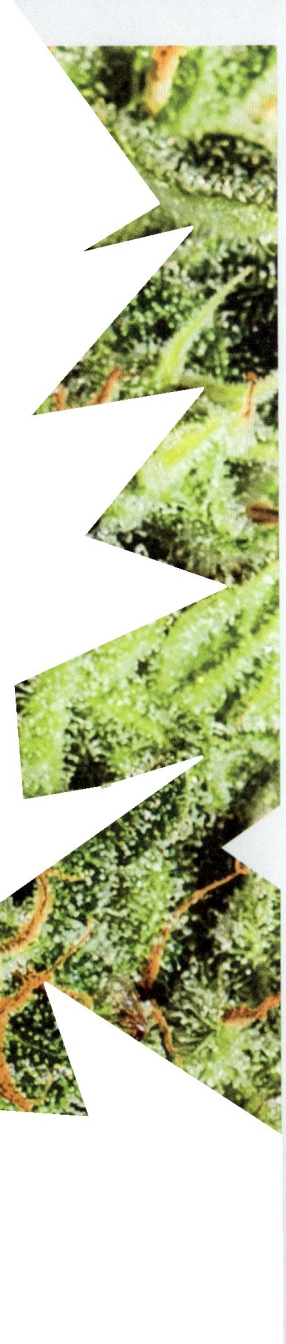

CHAPTER 6

Harvest Preparation:

Ideas for Harvest, Setting Up Your Drying Space, and Evaluating Ripeness

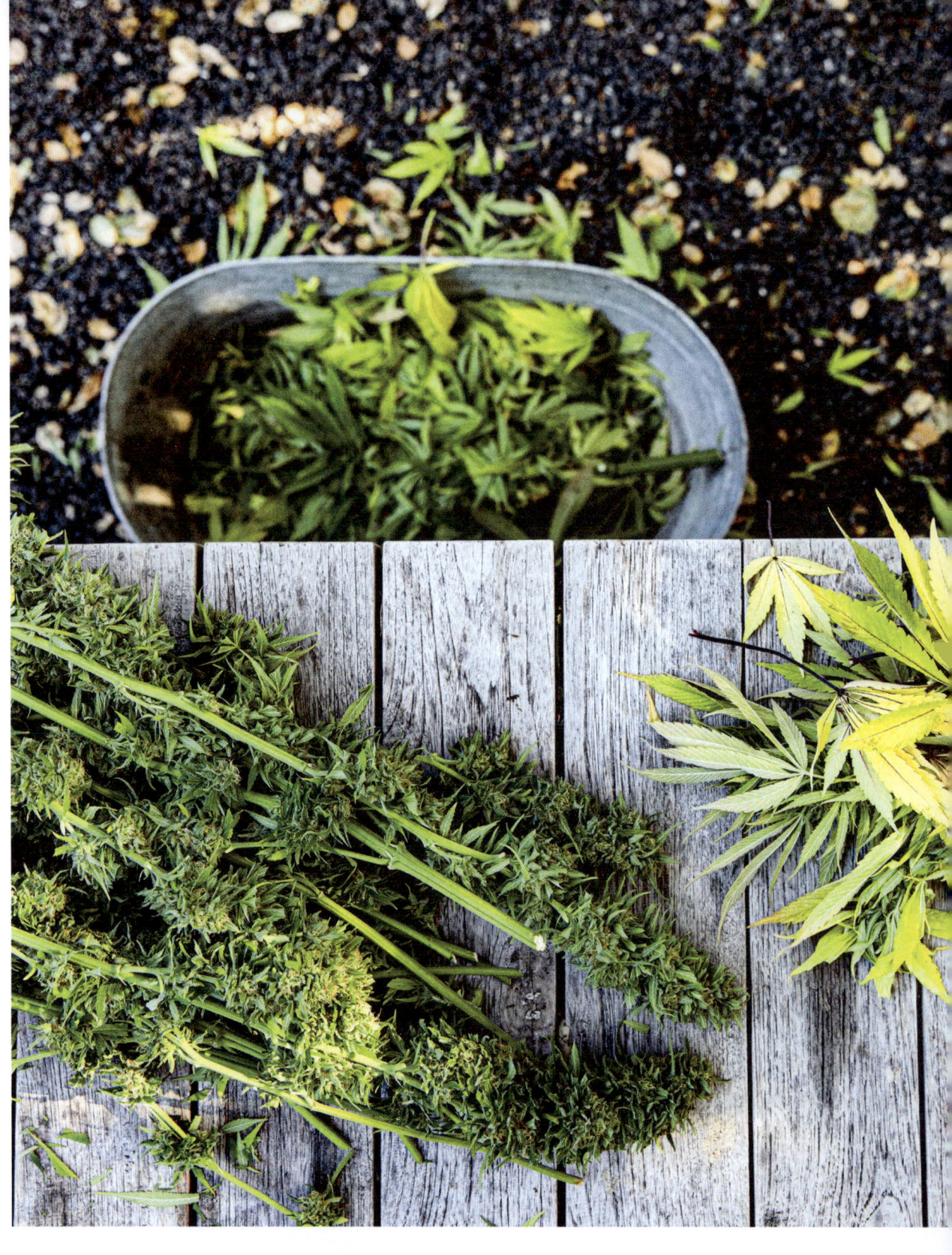

Finally—the moment you've been waiting for is here—it's time to harvest your grow. As your buds continue to grow and develop your plant will continue to reach taller, especially with cultivars that originated in warm climates. Use a magnifying glass to take a good long look at your flowers. Fall is just around the corner, which means it's almost the most thrilling time of year for the cannabis gardener—harvest time! The harvesting season is typically September 15 to November 1 for the Northern Hemisphere and March 15 to May 1 for the Southern Hemisphere. If you live in a tropical climate or grow auto-flowers, then your dates will be different. For tropical climates, the long season harvest time is the same as in temperate climates, whereas the short season harvest will be midwinter. Whether you've babied along one gorgeous lady in a planter or have a backyard full of big shrubby plants, it is a thrill to harvest your flower. If you're new to growing cannabis, knowing when and how to harvest can feel daunting. Do not fear, my friend—this chapter will guide you through harvesting your cannabis flower every step of the way, focusing on plant and flower changes and preparing your drying space. What you intend to create with your cannabis will also inform how you harvest; as such, it's important to understand how to gather the best of your plant to match what you're going to do with it. Your cannabis plant offers more than bud, and as a home cannabis gardener, you can enjoy the plant throughout the growing season. One of the fabulous benefits to growing your own is using parts of the plant both before and during harvest time in tisanes, smoothies, and bouquets. Here are some ideas for you to get the most your of your garden-grown weed.

WHAT TO HARVEST	IDEAS FOR USE	HOW TO STORE	NOTES
Bud—full size, dried and cured	Smoking, whole flower vaping, concentrates, edibles, and tinctures	Store dried, cured bud airtight in a cool, dark spot	Highest cannabinoid concentration is in your biggest, ripest bud. Suitable for most recipes (see chapter 8)
Bud—smaller bud, dried and cured	Tisanes, tinctures, concentrates, smoking, concentrates, and edibles	Store dried, cured bud airtight in a cool, dark spot	Potent little buds are wonderful to use in tinctures and edibles (see chapter 8)
Sugar leaves	Concentrates, edibles, tisanes	Store dried, cured sugar leaves airtight in a cool, dark spot	Less potent than bud, but still rich in cannabinoids and terpenes (see page 116)
Small leaves—dried	Tisanes, concentrates for topicals	Flash dry small leaves for tisane	Less potent than either bud or sugar leaves; brew delicious mellow tisane with dried leaves (see page 172)
Small leaves—fresh	Tisanes, smoothies, juices	Use fresh, freeze for future use	Less potent than either bud or sugar leaves; brew delicious mellow tisane (see page 172), excellent in juices and smoothies for THCa and CBDa (see page 15)
Fan leaves—fresh	Compost, smoothies, juices	Use fresh	Fan leaves are the least potent part of the edible cannabis plant, and are a healthy source of nutrients for juices and smoothies
Stems	Compost	Chop into chunks for the compost pile	
Roots	Compost, detoction	Dry for using in a detoction or chop up roots for the compost pile	Unique cannabinoids are found in cannabis root
Seed	Plant next spring	Store in a dry, cool, dark place	Free cannabis seeds for next year's grow (see page 97)

You're getting so close to picking your flowers, but before you do, choose the best place for drying your weed. Setting up a drying space before you start picking is important. Drying takes about two weeks—you'll feel as if you're living in an herbalist shop for those weeks, but it ends soon enough. There are four things that degrade harvested cannabis—light, oxygen (air), heat, and time—and these start to affect it the minute you pick your bud. The sun, which used to be your plant's lifeline of energy, is suddenly a threat to the potency and character of your grow. Temperature and humidity are the two most important factors to consider when drying your cannabis flower. The goal in setting up a drying space is to maximize potency and flavor of your weed. The ideal humidity in which to dry your weed is 45 to 55 percent, and the best temperature is between 65° and 70°F. Luckily, this temperature is pretty typical autumn weather for most of the temperate areas of the world.

Drying Space Supplies

Clothesline

Cotton string

Card stock and pen for labeling

Electric fan

Dehumidifier (only for humid environments)

Thermometer/hygrometer

30× Jeweler's loupe for examining trichomes

Inside or Out?

Your first decision will be to choose whether to set up your drying spot indoors or outside in a protected area. For most of us, inside is the best place to dry weed, since an inside area offers your harvested bud protection from direct sunlight, fluctuating temperatures, and inconsistent humidity or rain. You may live in areas with rainy weather, high winds, or heat waves—none of which is optimal for drying weed.

Let's explore the best spots in your apartment or house to dry your grow. Think about how each of your indoor spaces feels. In each one, there are microclimates, with some areas hotter and drier than others—attic vs basement, for example. Can you think of a spot with space enough to hang your 2- to 3-foot branch segments upside down and leave them undisturbed for about two weeks? Depending on the size of your plants, these segments can fill a small closet—or a whole bedroom if you grew several big plants.

If you live in a humid climate or will be drying your weed during a cold, wet time of year, you'll need to hang the branches inside to ensure the best conditions, a place where you can make sure there is good airflow to allow the cannabis flower to dry at a good rate—not too fast, not too slow. Use an electric fan to create a gentle, indirect airflow over all the hanging bud. You may need to invest in a dehumidifier if you expect to have persistently humid weather during the drying time. Not sure what your humidity is? I recommend purchasing a thermometer/hygrometer (a temperature and humidity sensor)—an inexpensive tool to help you monitor or select the best spots in your space for drying your weed.

If you grew more than one cultivar of cannabis, be prepared to label and group the drying branches together by type in the drying area. Each weed has its own drying speed, so it's efficient to group the drying weed by plant. Additionally, I like to keep track of how any one cultivar of cannabis affects me, so I find it helpful to keep harvested bud from each plant separated from bud of other plants, even if they are from the same named cultivar.

For the first several days of drying, your weed will be powerfully fragrant. And, as you can imagine, the more bud you have to dry, the more powerful the fragrance will be, so just a warning: be ready for the unique, amazingly strong scent of your cannabis as it dries. Take heart, though; the smells aren't very noticeable after the first week.

If you have strictly limited indoor space and happen to live in an area with mild, dry autumn weather, a shed or covered porch can be a fine spot to dry your weed—as long as you can secure the area. If you will be drying outside in the shade, the natural outdoor airflow should be fine for drying your branches at a measured pace. You will need, of course, to protect your drying cannabis from any rain or dew and from direct sunlight. And for those desert dwellers reading this, with your very arid climate, you can slow the rate of drying by dry trimming, or keeping some of the leaves on your drying bud (see page 126). Be creative and err on the side of the practical while drying. It may take over your limited indoor space for a while, but think of it as temporary—the whole drying process is usually complete in less than three weeks.

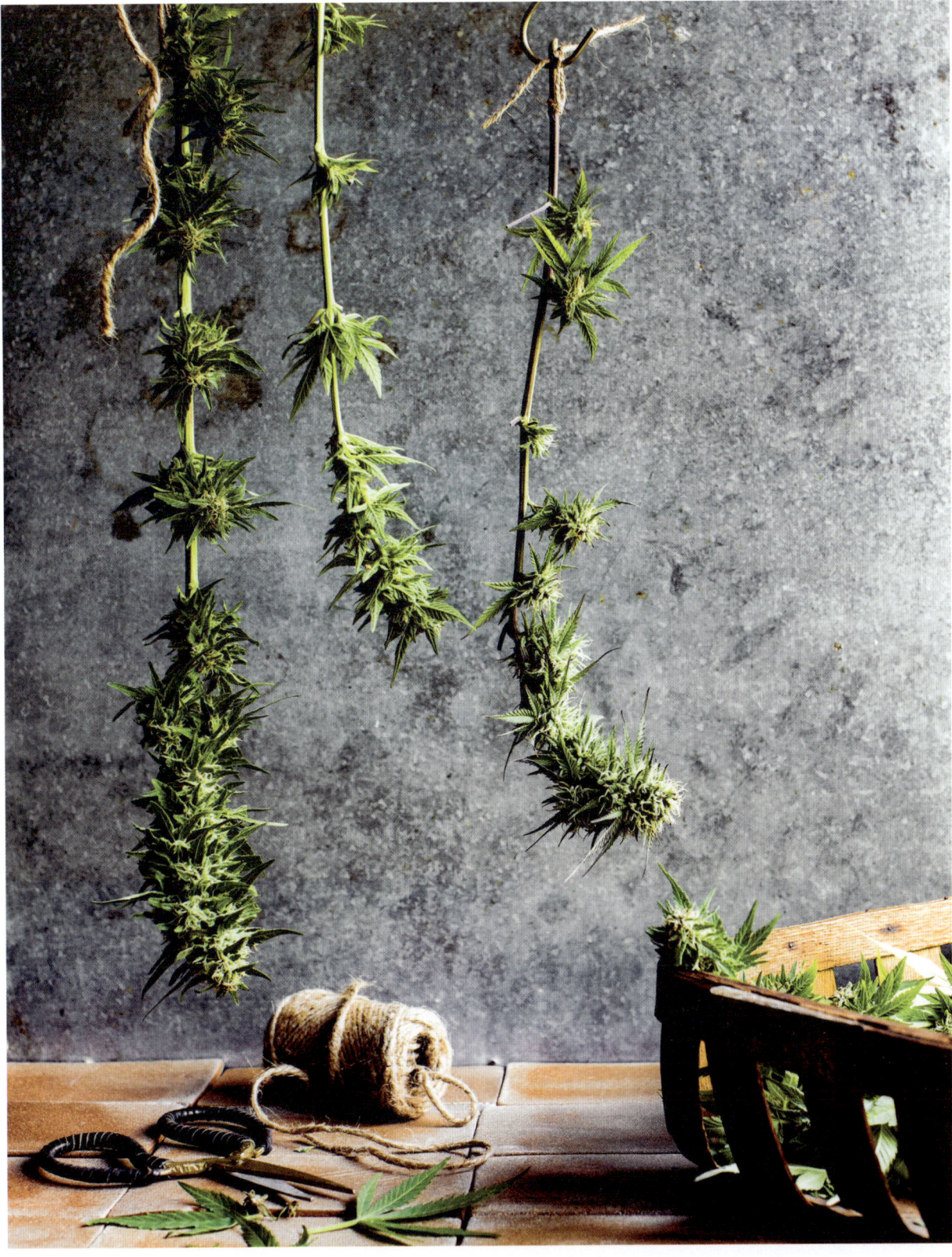

In my garden . . .

Where I grow, my garage is the best spot to dry my weed. The space is secure and dark, with enough room to hang several clotheslines. I use a small portable fan for gentle airflow. My weed remains out of the way of my day-to-day life—an important detail to consider for those of us living in small spaces. I could choose to take over a room inside my house, but since my home is petite, the smell of drying weed would be a tad overwhelming. Drying in the garage helps, too, to diffuse the smell, turning it into a pleasant waft rather than an olfactory barrage.

KNOWING WHEN TO PICK

Okay, friends. Now it's time for you to put on your detective hat and look for the clues that your plant is showing through its flowers—clues to indicate the best time to harvest. You've likely made decisions like this a number of times. If you've ever plucked a beautiful red tomato off a vine, then you've used clues from the fruit to tell you when it's ripe. You used your eyes, noticing the plump swell of the fruit, the change in color from green to bright red. You used your nose, inhaling the warm spicy scent of a tomato, to know that it was ripe. The process is similar when you're deciding whether your cannabis flowers are ready, but the signs are different. Your flowers will speak to you, and you need to learn their language to know what they're trying to tell you.

Changes to the Plant: Sugar Leaves, Fan Leaves, and Branch Support
As your plants enter late maturity, you will notice some changes. Here's what to look for.

Sugar leaves. As you look at your plant's colas (the cluster of buds at the very top of the plant), notice the sparkly little leaves crowded among the flowers. Sugar leaves are loaded with resins, almost as concentrated as the flower buds. They are found just beneath and nestled in the middle of the colas.

Fan leaves. The fan leaves (the large leaves extending out from the nodes) will be going through changes as your plant focuses its remaining energy on flower production. Your plant will stop making new big fan leaves as the flowering period enters its final stage. Some especially vigorous plants will retain all their fan leaves, and they will stay green and bright for the duration of flowering. However, most plants will show signs of fatigue as they give their all to the flowers. The oldest fan leaves, especially those in the shady interior of the plant, will yellow and fall off the plant. This is okay. Your plants are preparing to die; they know what they're doing by conserving resources and concentrating on flower production. Look for any powdery mildew and remove any infected leaves. If you discover powdery mildew and still have a week or more to go before flowering finishes, consider treating the remaining plant to keep the leaves going until the flowers are mature (see page 105). If you notice a sudden yellowing of leaves in more than just the oldest leaves or if the yellowing leaves of an entire branch are involved, it may be time for some intervention. If a whole branch shows problems, you may have a fungal infection on that branch. Check out the buds on the affected branch and inspect the colas for bud rot (see page 106).

Branch support. Finally, inspect your plant's stems—especially where lateral branches connect with the main stem. They should feel sturdy and whole—with no signs of rotting or weakness. Cannabis stalks are remarkably strong and flexible due to the long, resilient fibers in the stalks; historically, one of the most important uses for cannabis was for making fabric and rope. Give your branch a gentle shake—how heavy does it seem? You should be able to tell intuitively whether or not your plant's branches seem stable and strong enough to complete the flowering period. If you think that the branch won't be able to hold up the flower, offer additional support with a stake for any weak or particularly heavy branches. It never hurts to stake your plant at this stage of development, so if you're undecided about providing additional support, just go for it. Finally—check the weather forecast. An incoming storm can knock over plants with heavy ripe colas. Be sure that your plants are supported in case a windy rainstorm threatens before you've picked all of your flower.

Changes to the Flowers
It's such a joy to see the cannabis flowers emerge and ripen. Each cola is a dense clump of many individual flowers—more than a hundred in the largest colas.

If you've been paying attention to the growing colas on your plant, you will notice that they are different sizes and are named according to where you find them on the plant. Stand back and take a good look at your plant,

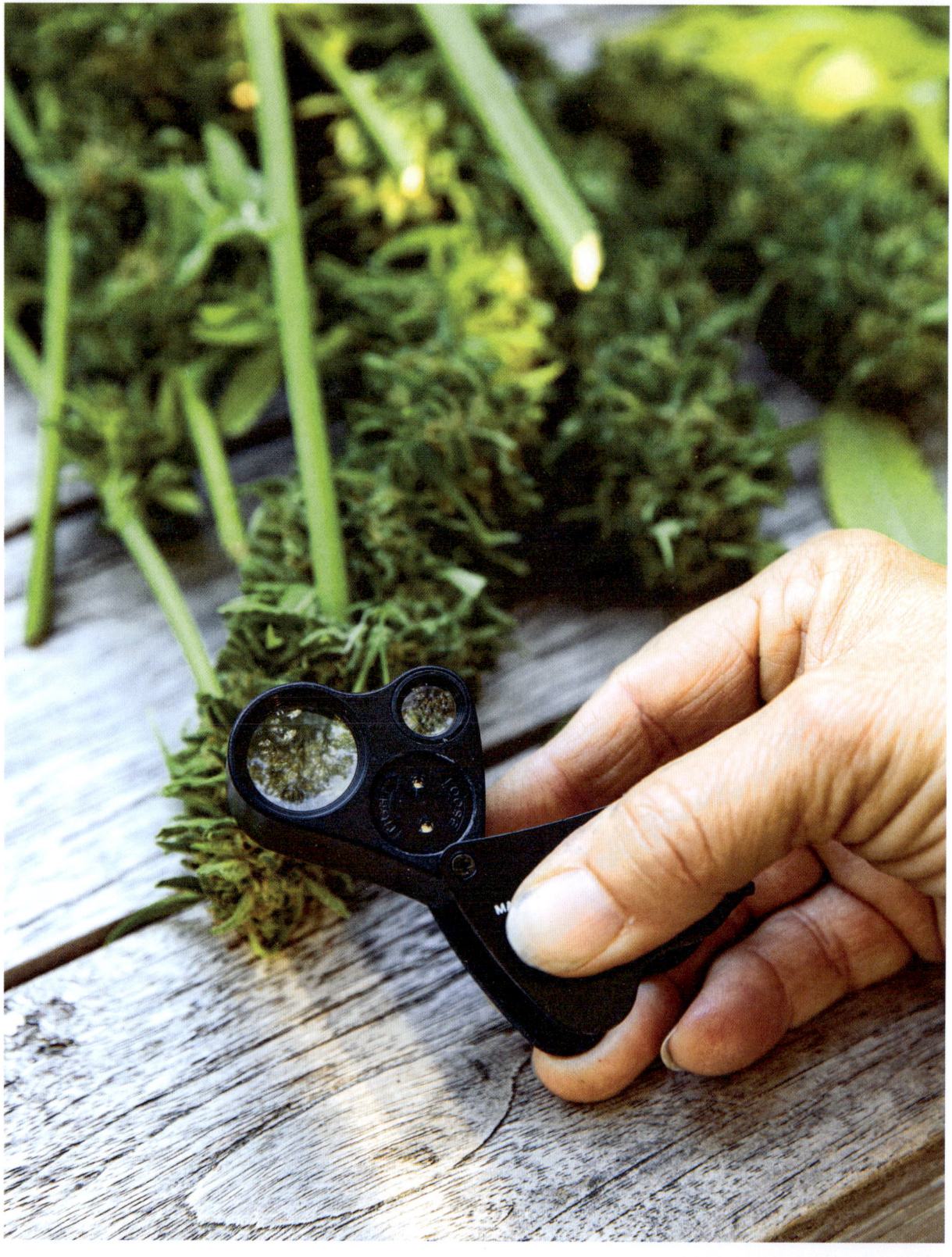

starting at the top. The topmost, or apical, cola is the largest on the plant and is likely to ripen first. If you pinched back your plant when it was little, you may not have one apical cola but rather two or more. No matter—the highest-growing colas will be the biggest. The next largest colas—the secondary colas—grow on large lateral branches that are lower on the plant. Tertiary colas, or popcorn colas, are smaller yet. You'll find them located on the smallest branch tips and on the inside of the plant. You may discover that these popcorn colas ripen days or even weeks later than the bigger colas. After you've picked the big buds, these little ones will get more sun and ripen to their full potential.

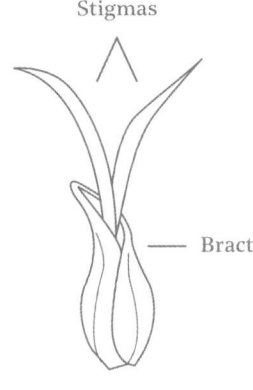

THE FEMALE FLOWER

Stigmas and trichomes are the two best signs of bud ripeness. Pay attention to these two structures and you will know when to pick your bud. The goal is to pick your fully mature female flower when it is at its peak of readiness: the buds are sparkly and sticky and smell powerfully fragrant when lightly brushed with your finger. Your flower buds will feel firm but not hard. Some cannabis has dense, chunky colas, while others have fluffier ones. Don't get too caught up in the denseness of the bud—focus on trichomes and stigmas for signs of ripeness.

Stigmas

To view the stigmas, look closely at the cola and locate a single flower—each single female cannabis flower is small, ¼ to ½ inch long. The flower can be described as looking like a lentil-size green bulb with two feathery, straight antenna-like structures emerging from the bulb. The bulbous portion of the flower is made up of an ovule covered by two trichome-covered bracts. Stigmas are the specialized structures that are designed to capture pollen. When your female cannabis plants unfurl their stigmas, they can become fertilized if there are any mature male cannabis plants in the area. The stigmas emerge from the ovule straight and pale. As the bud ages and ripens, there will be visible changes to the stigmas. When you notice some of the stigmas drying, becoming curled and darker in color, this is a sign that the flower colas are reaching peak ripeness. *At maturity, the stigmas shrivel, curl, and darken. This is an important clue to help you know when to pick your weed.*

Trichomes

It's truly amazing to see your flowers shine in bright sunlight, looking as if they are covered in diamond dust. This sparkle is caused by the thick blanket of trichomes on the flower bud and sugar leaves. Many plants make trichomes, but cannabis is the trichome champ of the plant world. Using a 30× jeweler's loupe, examine the glittery covering on each hirsute (fuzzy) flower and sugar leaf. This covering is a riot of luminous trichomes, packed with cannabinoids and terpenes. When magnified, trichomes look like tiny, shiny, skinny stemmed mushrooms. You will notice that some of them are clear, some may be slightly cloudy white, some may be yellow or amber. This trichome color change offers vital clues as to flower maturity. When trichomes first emerge, they are clear. With time, the trichomes turn cloudy, then white, and finally settle into amber before desiccating and falling off. At maturity, your bud's trichomes will likely be a combination of clear, cloudy, white, and amber. *When most of the trichomes are milky white, your flower is at peak ripeness.* Trichomes on past-the-prime bud are dark and shriveled. Each cola matures at a slightly different time from its neighboring branches, so inspect each one carefully until you gain confidence and experience in choosing ripeness. Generally, those colas that are in the most sunshine will ripen first. Flowers change throughout the day, with cannabinoid and terpene levels waxing and waning according to the time. The cannabinoid and terpene levels are at their highest during the morning, so harvest earlier in the day for ideal flower conditions. The time of day when you pick is less important than the overall ripeness of the bud, but nonetheless, it's something to consider.

Ripening Stages

You may find that your weed ripens over a couple of weeks. If you have more than one cultivar growing in your garden, they will likely have different ripening times. Ripeness is on a continuum, or a bell curve. Harvest in the home garden extends over the course of a week or more, especially if you have a couple different types of cannabis growing. Take your time with the harvest, and enjoy the process.

Early stage. The trichomes are full size and clear, the flower buds are sparkly, and stigmas are beginning to shrivel and darken. This is the early stage, and the flower buds are still maturing toward full expression of their cannabinoids. If you are forced to harvest your plant at the early ripeness stage, it's okay. Your bud will be less potent but still good. Sometimes you will make the call to harvest early due to a forecast of snow, freezing temperatures, or rainy, windy weather. If your plant was attacked by bud rot, you may need to harvest early to save what you can.

Peak stage. The buds are dense and sparkly, and most of the trichomes are milky white. A few trichomes are clear, and a few are amber. Most of the stigmas are shriveled and darkened. This is the peak of ripeness and the best time to pick for the full expression of cannabinoids and terpenes—the best potency and flavor.

Late stage. The trichomes are mostly yellowing or amber, with some milky white. Stigmas are uniformly shriveled and dark. This is late in the bud-picking stage. You will have an overall less-potent product, with some of the THCa transformed into THC, then CBN. In high-CBD varieties, overly mature bud will express less CBDa, having transformed it into CBD. Better late than never—just get it all picked and drying as soon as possible.

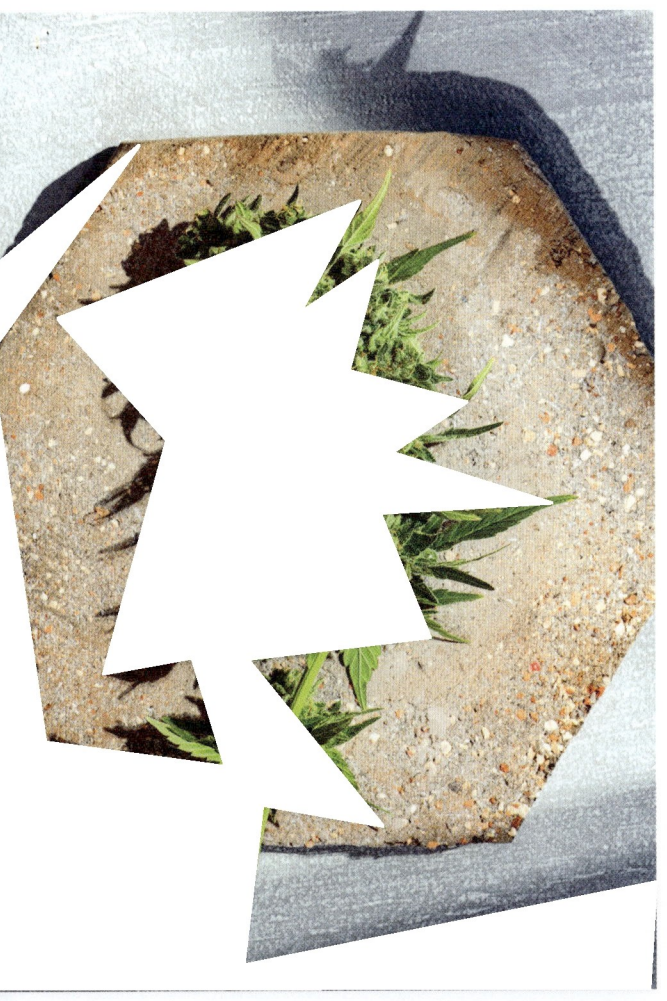

Don't fret about choosing the perfect moment to pick. If you've been paying attention to your flower, inspected the trichomes with your loupe, and seen the shriveled stigmas, use your best guess and pick. Each harvest brings with it an opportunity for you to learn and grow as a gardener. Don't let perfect be the enemy of good. Remember to enjoy yourself. I like to brew up a pot of freshly harvested cannabis bud tisane with the first cut of the harvest (see page 172). I bring my steaming mug with me to my little garden and sip while I do some trimming. I like to think it helps me connect to the plant as I get a waft of the tasty terpenes, appreciating the unique fragrance and flavor it offers.

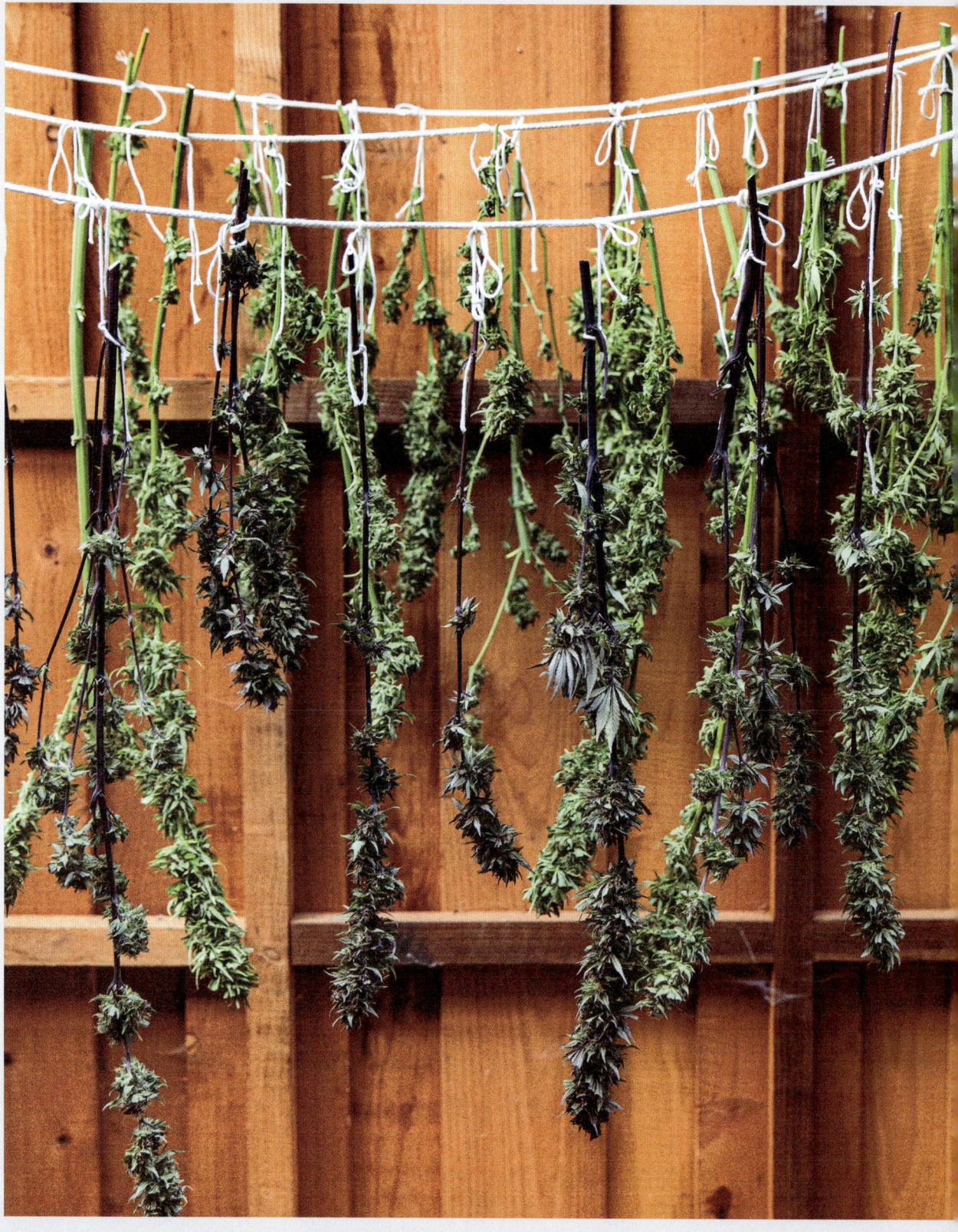

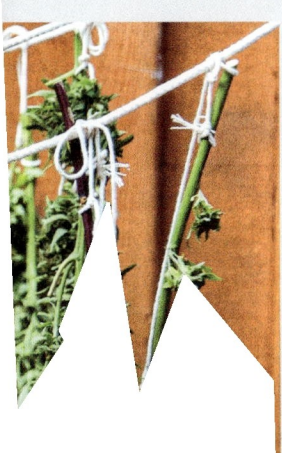

CHAPTER 7

Time to Harvest:

Picking, Trimming, Drying, Curing, and Storing Your Grow

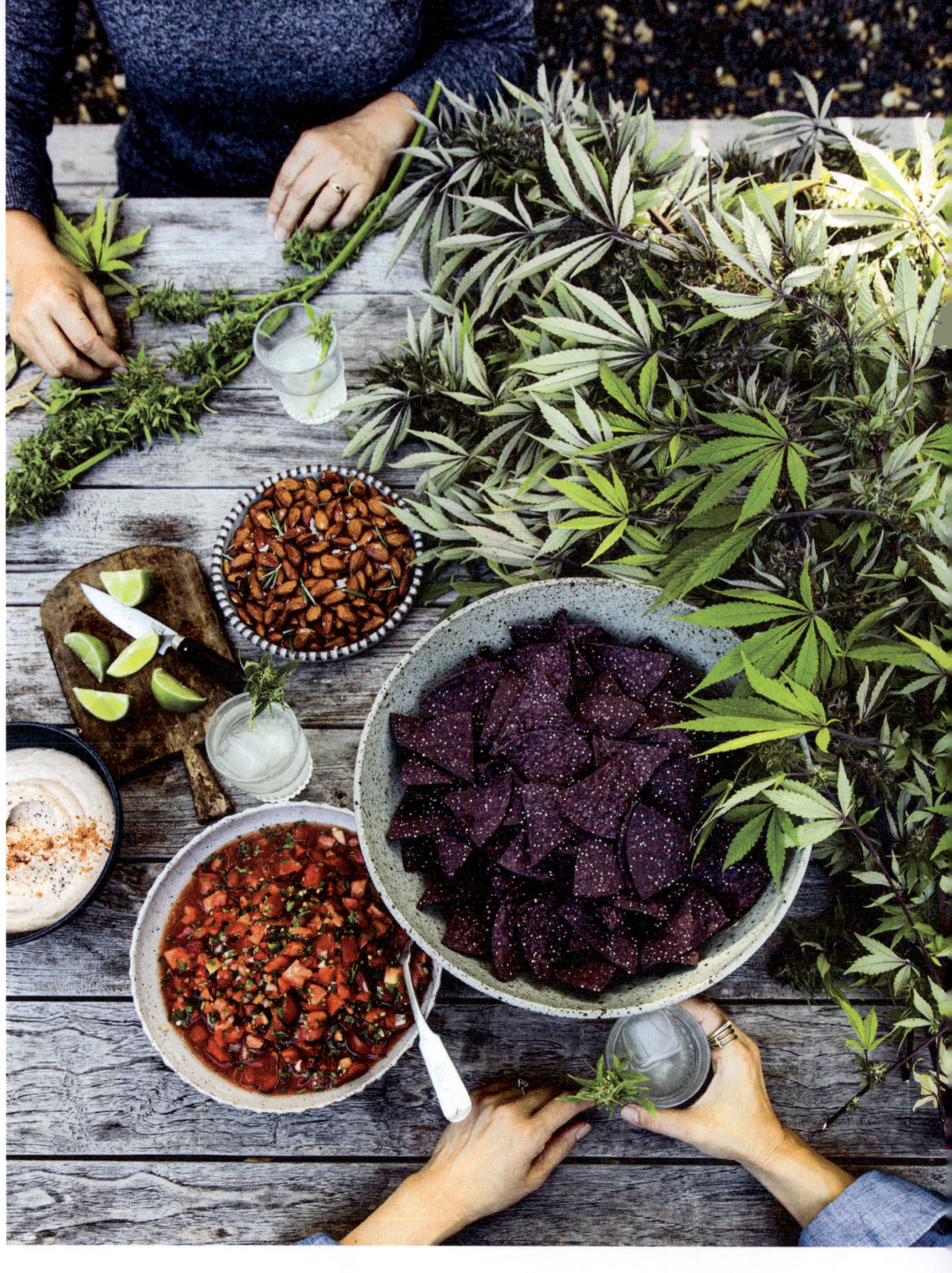

You've set up your drying space, your flowers are ripe—now comes the fun part. Harvesting your home grow involves three things: cutting branches, removing unwanted leaves, and hanging the trimmed branches in your drying space. As mentioned in chapter 6, knowing what you want to do with your grow before you start picking is very helpful, especially for your first harvest. Consider how you'd like to make the most of your plant before you start harvesting, and you'll have a happier time cutting, trimming, and hanging your weed. Take a look at the table on page 112, or peek at the ideas for using your harvest in chapter 8 for some pre-harvest inspiration.

Harvest can take several days, perhaps weeks, depending on how evenly your flower ripens. Sun-grown weed is going to have several different sizes of colas (bud clusters). The topmost (apical) cola is the largest—and with its head in the sunny sky, it's likely to ripen first. The next largest colas will be found on the ends of the large lateral branches and will ripen at about the same time as the apical cola. The smaller colas toward the center of the plant will likely ripen days to weeks later. One of the luxuries of being a home grower is that you can pick your colas when they are ready, not when you can hire trimmers. If you have one beautiful cannabis plant, you will be able to cut and trim in an afternoon or so. More plants will take more time—especially if you have big bushy grows. And if you decided to go for it this year with a garden full of monster plants, you may need some help. If so, consider making this a social event. Have a trim party—you will likely be a very popular host. Invite some of your trusted friends, arm them with trimmers, spin some tunes, set out some snacks and drinks, and make a party out of it. The only thing better than connecting with your plants is to include your friends and family in the joy! Send your friends home with a couple branches to dry and use for themselves as a thank-you for their efforts. It's the ultimate win-win: you get help harvesting, your friends get a little stash, and everyone has a good time connecting with the plant universe.

Supplies You Will Need

Clothesline or wooden dowel for hanging

Cotton string

Disposable gloves (optional)

Fan

Jeweler's loupe (30× or 60×)

Glass jars with lids or Grove Bags

Magnifying glass (5× or 10×)

Mesh herb-drying bag (optional)

Olive oil and kosher salt

Handheld pruner

Rags

Rubbing alcohol

Labels (optional)

Large bowls

Trimmers: 1 for each person trimming

Viewing scope (optional)

. . . and friends and snacks (optional—but more fun!)

WET AND DRY TRIMMING

Trimming is the process of removing leaves from the cut cannabis branches. Trimming is a key step in harvesting your weed, with two main methods of trimming: wet trim and dry trim. Either method can work; each has pros and cons.

Wet trimming means that you remove all of the leaves from your flower bud branches before hanging them up to dry. One of the reasons why folks wet trim is to minimize mold growth on the drying bud. Removing the overlying leaves from the bud increases the airflow around the flowers and decreases moisture levels quickly. Wet trimming allows you to separate the sugar leaves from the bud before drying. I like to quick-dry some of the sugar leaves for herbal tisanes (see page 172), and wet trimming gives me abundant sugar leaves to quick-dry and store airtight. Another reason to wet trim is to consolidate most of the harvest labor into one period.

Dry trimming means to remove unwanted leaves from your branches after they have been hung and dried. Dry trimming is a great idea for those of you living in arid climates or if you need to dry your weed outside. In very arid climates, with ambient humidity of 30 percent or less, bud will dry too quickly, with a loss of terpenes and cannabinoids. Leaving some leaves on the branches while they are drying allows the bud to dry at a measured pace. Dry trimming is also a great idea if you are pressed for time during the peak harvest window. Perhaps your colas decide to get 100 percent ripe just as a storm is coming—time to harvest those branches and worry about trimming later. If you are new to cannabis growing, I recommend trying out both wet trimming and dry trimming methods to see which one works best for you.

HOW TO CUT AND TRIM CANNABIS

It's helpful to get organized before you begin cutting and trimming. Set up a workstation with plenty of space for the freshly picked branches. A picnic table or a folding table and chairs for each trimmer will work well. If you don't have access to an outdoor table and are comfortable sitting on the ground, then lay a drop cloth or tarp on the ground to serve as your workstation. If you'll be collecting leaves for use in salves, tinctures, and edibles, be sure to have bowls or buckets to keep them separate from the trimmed branches. Cannabis branches are bulky, so if the space on your table is at a premium, set out an old tablecloth on the ground to keep the cut branches dirt-free as they wait to be trimmed. Trimming inside the house is perfectly fine, too—just remember that the smell becomes potent as the trimming proceeds.

STEP ONE | Cutting Branches

It's important to cut, trim, and hang your branches in one day. You risk damaging the trichomes or encouraging mold if you leave your cut branches in a pile for more than that. If you are pressed for time, cut only as many branches as you can trim and hang in one sitting. It's better to keep your flower on the plant—and fresh—rather than cut and lying in a pile. Start by cutting several branches with ripe cola(s), leaving a couple of inches of stem to tie the string onto. It's up to you to decide where to cut any given branch—there is no perfect length. The important thing is to cut a section that has ripe bud. In my experience, most of the branch pieces I cut tend to be between 1 and 3 feet in length. At the end of the harvest, I usually have some small later-ripening buds to pick on smaller branchlets. Stay focused on your goal of collecting only ripe flower buds and you can't mess up. Mound the branches in the center of the trimming table. Branch by branch, inspect the fan leaves. Remove any yellowing or diseased-looking leaves, setting those aside for the compost pile or greens recycling bin.

STEP TWO | Removing Bud Rot and Debris

Next, thoroughly inspect your colas for bud rot and remove any rotten bits. Bud rot will be obvious—it will be tan or gray-brown and crumbly. You'll need to examine the flower buds with your eyes, then with your fingers. Like a cavity in your tooth, most of the damage will be beneath the surface of the flower area, so you'll need to probe. Remove any infected parts and discard them. Don't worry—the rest of the cola that looks healthy is just fine and will dry nicely. Sometimes you'll need to cut a dense cola apart if there is bud rot in the center. As long as you trim away the diseased parts, you're good to go—dry any flower pieces in a mesh herb-drying bag if you can't easily attach a string for hanging. If you see any pieces of debris or insect remains, brush them off with your fingers or, as a last resort, give the cola a gentle dip in clean water—but only very quickly. Your goal is to dry your buds before mold can set in, and water-soaked buds will be more prone to getting moldy in the drying stage.

STEP THREE | Trimming

Healthy green fan leaves can be set aside for concentrates (see page 156). If you're dry trimming, remove just the fan leaves and any smaller leaves that are yellowing or diseased and you're done with trimming. For those of you who are wet trimming, you have a few more cuts to make. Remove and set aside any healthy-looking small leaves for tisanes (see page 172); I usually save leaves that are between 3 and 5 centimeters for this use. Leave the tiny sugar leaves—loaded with trichomes—on the branches or remove and save them for concentrates and tinctures or for drying for special tisanes (page 175). You will now be left with mostly leaf-less colas. You will notice that there are some tiny, spiky leaflets that remain in the nugs. Since I use much of my flower for high-quality tinctures and salves, I don't remove these—leaving my buds a little shaggy looking. If you are a fan of clean-shaven nugs for your pipe or bong, go ahead and trim the tiny spiky leaflets around your flower. This is also a wise practice if you have had any recent rain or if you have more humid than ideal drying conditions. After the first bunch of colas are processed, stop and assess the ripeness of the remaining flower. If it's ripe, it's time to move on to the smaller colas. These are the numerous colas that grow on lateral, interior branches of the plant. Trim these the same way as you did your main cola. Last of all, pick the smallest colas, the ones located on the smallest branch tips and deep on the inside of the plant. You may find that these ripen later (days or even weeks) than the bigger colas. After you've picked the big buds, these little guys will get more sun and ripen to their full potential. Because these little guys don't have much stem attached, I dry

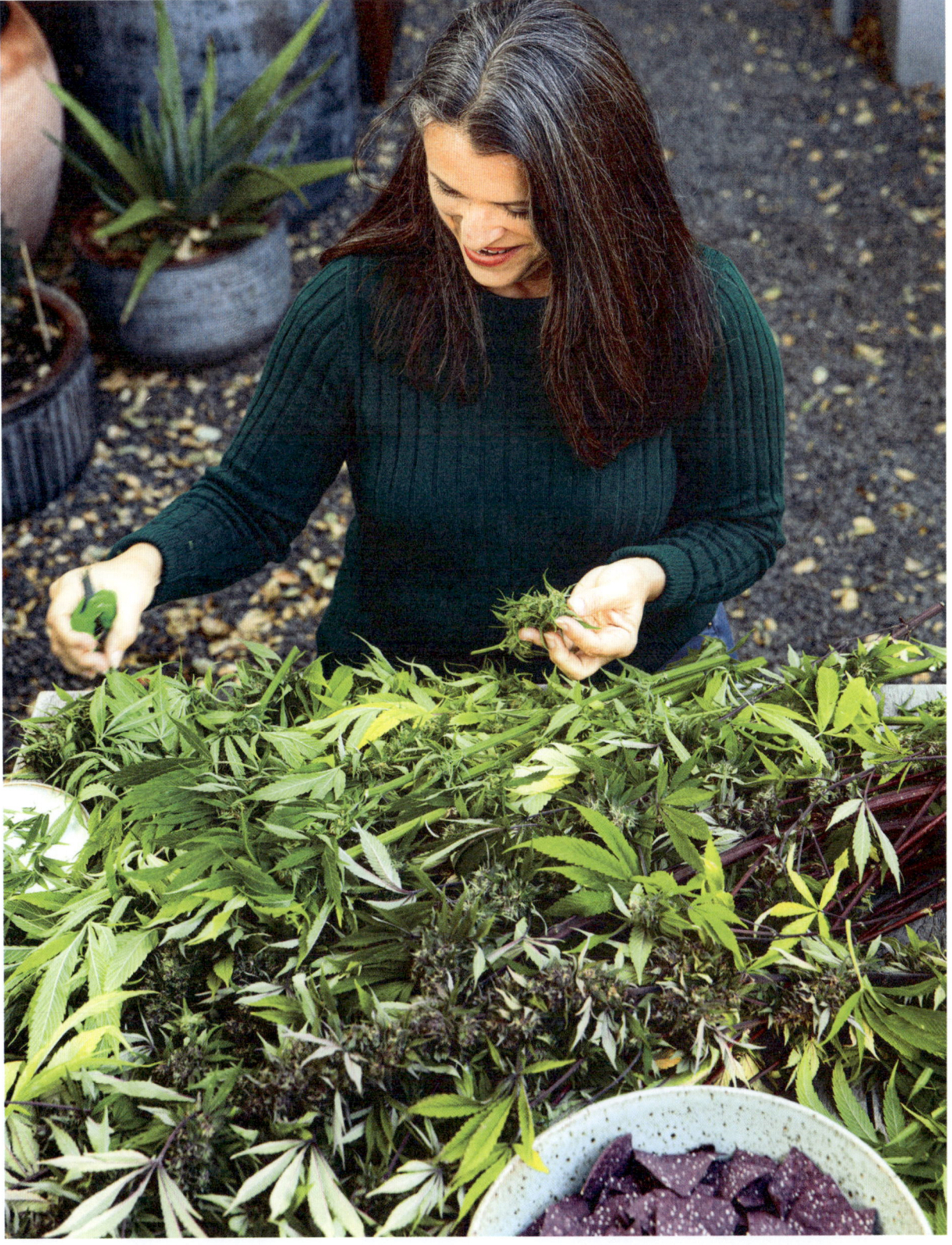

them in a mesh herb-drying bag. These are ideal to use to make concentrates for topicals (see page 159).

STEP FOUR | Hanging Up Your Trimmed Branches

After you've trimmed the branches to your liking, it's time to hang them up in your drying area. For brevity, I'll use my method—the clothesline—in the remaining description. I like to use cotton kitchen string to tie my trimmed branches to a clothesline. Not only is cotton kitchen string inexpensive, it's also compostable, making cleanup easier when I take the dried bud off the branches at the end of the drying stage. Stems and string just get composted—easy. To hang your stems up, cut a foot-long piece of string and use it to tie two equal-size branches together at their cut ends, leaving an inch or so of stem above the knot. Tent the two branches over the clothesline upside down, one branch on each side of the line, allowing gravity to hold them in place. You can also attach each stem separately to the clothesline, tying each with its own piece of cotton string. Leave at least an inch between branches to give your bud good airflow.

STEP FIVE | Clean Up

After trimming a few branches, you may notice that your trimmers and hands are getting sticky with resin. This is totally normal—and a sign of the quality of your weed. In fact, that sticky resin is hash. If you've chosen to wear disposable gloves, you can replace the gloves as needed. I usually trim with bare hands, since I prefer to feel the plant material as I trim. Whether or not you wear gloves, your trimmers will get gummy after a while. I recommend periodically cleaning off your trimmer blades with rubbing alcohol and a rag to remove the sticky resin and restore the smooth

Cleaning Resin Off Your Hands

To clean your skin, I recommend the olive oil and salt method. Pour a teaspoon or so of olive oil into your hand and sprinkle on some kosher salt. Scrub the olive oil and salt together, all over the sticky areas of your skin—especially on the finger pads. Wash off the oil and salt with warm water and hand soap. Rinse well and dry off your hands. And a bonus? Your hands will feel fabulous—smooth, exfoliated, moisturized.

cutting surface of your trimmer. You can clean your hands with rubbing alcohol as well, but this can be drying to the skin (see sidebar).

DRYING YOUR GROW

Drying your cannabis is simple: provide the right conditions and then wait, inspect, and relax. The goal is to provide a moderate pace of drying to preserve terpenes and cannabinoids, avoid mold growth, and achieve a smooth, flavorful bud to smoke or use in other preparations. The chlorophyll in the flower will disappear, causing your flower and branches to go from bright green to dull green. The fresh, strong odor of cut weed will continue to radiate from the grow room for a couple of days, moving from powerfully fragrant to pleasantly herbal. What you will be smelling is terpenes—glorious, fragrant terpenes. The terpenes in your plant are a group of compounds that have a range of weights that correspond directly to their volatility. The lightest, most volatile terpenes will evaporate most readily, with the heavier terpenes remaining in the bud. For this reason, your flower's finished fragrance will depend both on the cultivar you grew and on drying conditions. If your flower dries too quickly, you risk losing terpenes.

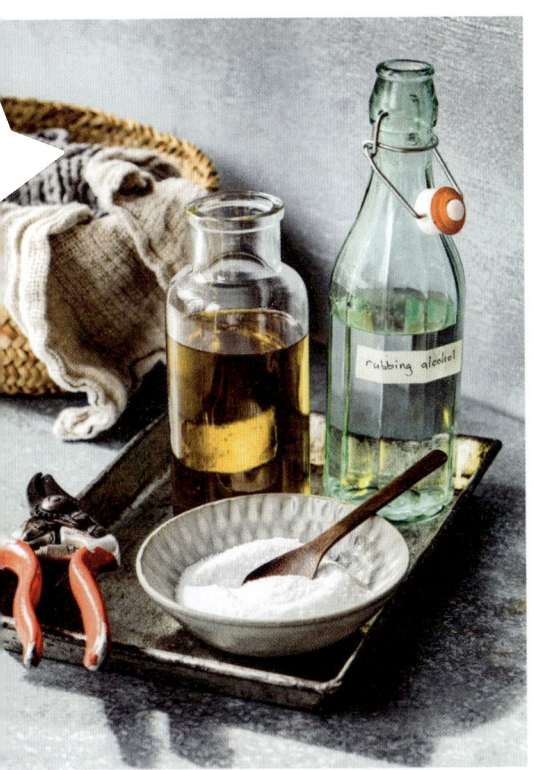

I recommend monitoring the drying bud daily, being sure there is no mold growth on the flower, especially on the big dense colas. If you have a thermometer/hygrometer, place it in the drying space and use this information to check the drying conditions for your harvest. If the humidity levels are in the ideal range of 45 to 55 percent, you should have nicely dried weed in two weeks or so. If ambient humidity levels are higher, 70 percent or more, be sure to provide constant but gentle airflow. Fans are particularly important if you're drying indoors, since there is little natural air circulation inside. Those living in very humid climates may wish to use a dehumidifier to control humidity in the drying space. To preserve the integrity of the trichomes on the buds, it's important to have gentle, direct airflow. How's the temperature in your drying room? If you are comfortable, then so are your flowers. The ideal drying temperature is around 65°F to 75°F. Cooler temperatures will slow drying, and higher temperatures will speed it up. As your flowers dry, the trichomes will become more brittle and fragile, so keep them on the bud and disturb them as little as possible with strong airflow or too much handling. If you see some moldy patches, trim those areas and increase the airflow.

As your plants finish ripening, continue to hang the newly ripe and trimmed branches in the drying area, being careful to keep track of when you hung the branches. Every so often after the first week, test the dryness of the branches. Notice the tiny leaves—they should be dry, with some of them brittle and others still pliable. The flowers will be somewhat less dense in their clusters, showing a little space between each clump. If you give your flower colas a close inspection with good light, you'll see that the stigmas are all shriveled and dry, darkened to their final hue. If you shine a bright light on the flowers and look with your jeweler's loupe, you should still see dense shiny trichomes on the flower surfaces—the goal!

CURING YOUR WEED

Curing is the next step in quality bud processing. Curing gives your bud time to readjust moisture levels throughout the bud while preserving terpenes and cannabinoids for maximum usability. Enzymatic changes are still happening in your flower bud, helping to create a smooth, pleasant flavor in the smokable bud. Proper drying and curing also set you up for the longest-lasting flower as well. How will you know when your cannabis

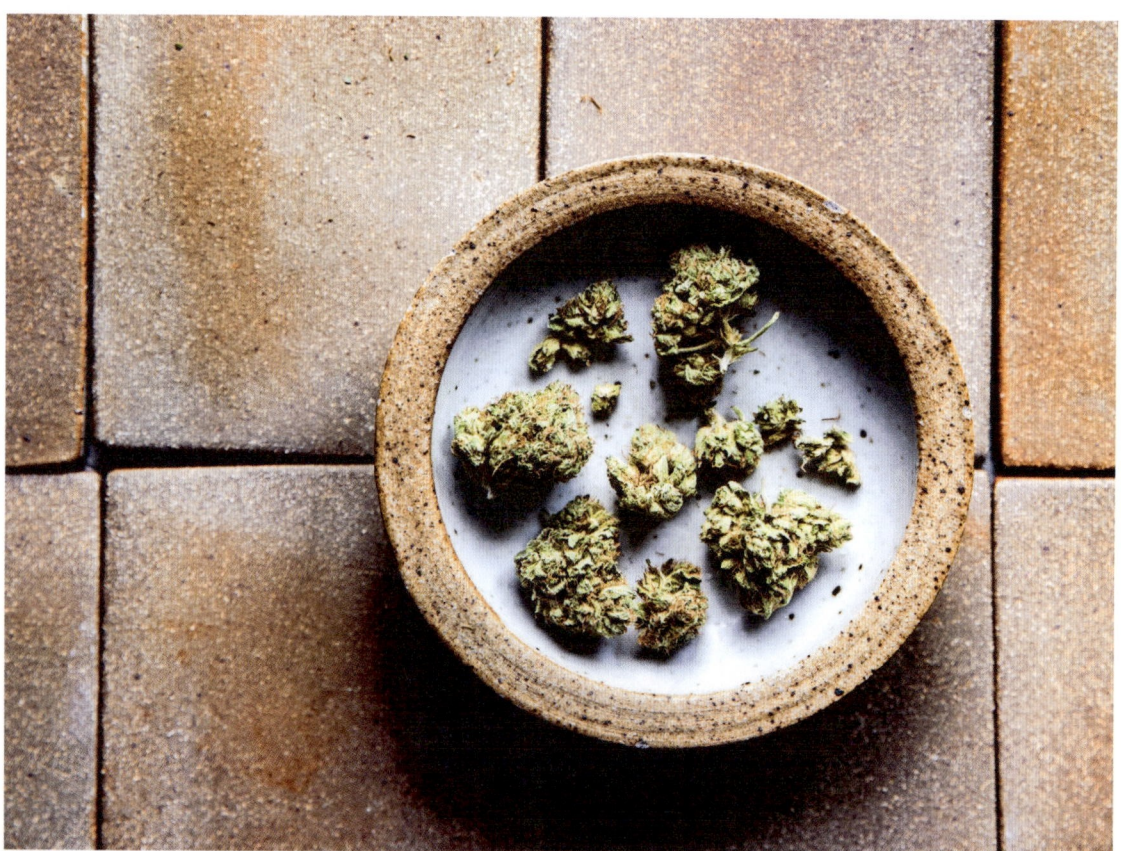

is done drying? When the small branches snap rather than bend. The buds should be dry to the touch on the outside but with a springy give from the inside. Now it's time to cure your dried weed.

Prepare Your Containers

To get your dry bud ready to cure, start by preparing your final storage receptacles. You will also need pruning shears to cut off the buds from the branches. I recommend that you invest in a set of large canning jars. I love to use half-gallon glass canning jars to store my bud. Because outdoor plants can be prolific, I find that the size of these airtight, reusable jars is efficient at holding a lot of weed. These jars are inexpensive, readily available, and useful for any storage needs when they aren't filled with cannabis bud. Any size jar is good—just be sure to get enough jars to hold all the bud that your lovely sun-blessed plants have so lavishly produced. There are some new cannabis-specific storage bags available, such as Grove Bags. These look like black plastic bags, but they are different from the typically available polypropylene bags sold for kitchen use. Grove Bags are specifically designed to resist the movement of terpenes and cannabinoids through the bag's walls, and so are a good choice if you don't want to use glass jars. Regular kitchen plastic storage bags are *not* a good option to store your cannabis for any length of time, because they are permeable to terpenes.

Packing for the Cure

Once you've done the snap test and have determined that your flower is nicely dried, it's time to get the bud cut off and into jars. Using pruners, snip the buds off the branches, and chop up the larger bud colas into chunks for best storage. Of course, if you have a fabulously huge intact cola, feel free to dry and cure it whole—great for show-and-tell and bragging rights at your next party. ("No way—you grew that bud? Sweet!") Lightly pack the dried bud into your final receptacle, either glass jars or cannabis-specific storage bags, to retain its normal shape. The bud should fill the whole container, with no headspace in the jar. If they are packed too tight, this may encourage mold growth, too loose and they'll lose terpenes to oxidation. When you've filled up a jar, screw on the lid and place the jar in a cool, dark spot.

The curing process has now begun and will continue for a month or so. The first several days are the most important. Every day for one week, open up your jars and give them a nice sniff. What do you notice? You should smell cannabis—but not mold. As you remove the jar to smell the curing weed, take a look at the inside of the lid. It should be dry, without any condensed moisture. If you do notice any moisture, that's a sign that your cannabis wasn't done drying and needs a bit more time outside the jar. To correct this problem, gently spread out the cut bud on a piece of raised mesh, such as a baking rack. After another couple of days, repack the bud in the jar and start curing again. I've never had a problem with moisture retention, but it's always good to check. After the first several days of monitoring your bud, the curing process will proceed with success. Continue to open up your airtight glass storage jars for a minute every couple of days to release moisture and gasses. And take time to enjoy the fruits of your gardening: can you believe that you grew this? So amazing. The fragrance should be delicious, rich, and unique for each cultivar of cannabis. After a month, your weed is basically stable and cured. Time to properly store your harvest— and enjoy it.

Storing: Controlling Oxygen, Light, Heat, and Time

Dried, cured bud will gradually change over time, and the goal of good storage is to slow this natural rate of change. Oxygen, light, heat, and time are the enemies of your bud. Why? These are factors that cause degradation of cannabinoids and terpenes in your dried, cured flower. Cannabinoids change over time by spontaneously decarboxylating (see page 140). When exposed to air, terpenes are sensitive to oxidation and evaporation, natural biochemical processes that degrade the quality of your dried bud. It is important to keep the dried bud fragrant and potent for as long as possible, and you do this by controlling the oxygen, light, and temperature conditions for your flower. You can't control time, but you can minimize the impact of the other three factors. Once you've properly dried and cured your weed, aim to preserve the bud's quality for best flavor and potency.

Store your weed in airtight containers in a cool, dark spot. A basement, garage, or closet are good choices. If you choose to freeze your dried bud, be sure to bring it to room temp before opening the container for use. Your weed will stay fresh for at least a year if properly dried, cured, and stored. Bud that is stored for longer than that will remain useful, but the cannabinoid profile will slowly change over time. Now you can relax and enjoy some of your home grow. You've connected with the earth, with the plant kingdom, and with the cannabis community in a deeper way. I hope you enjoyed your experience and learned from it—and took notes for a better grow next year.

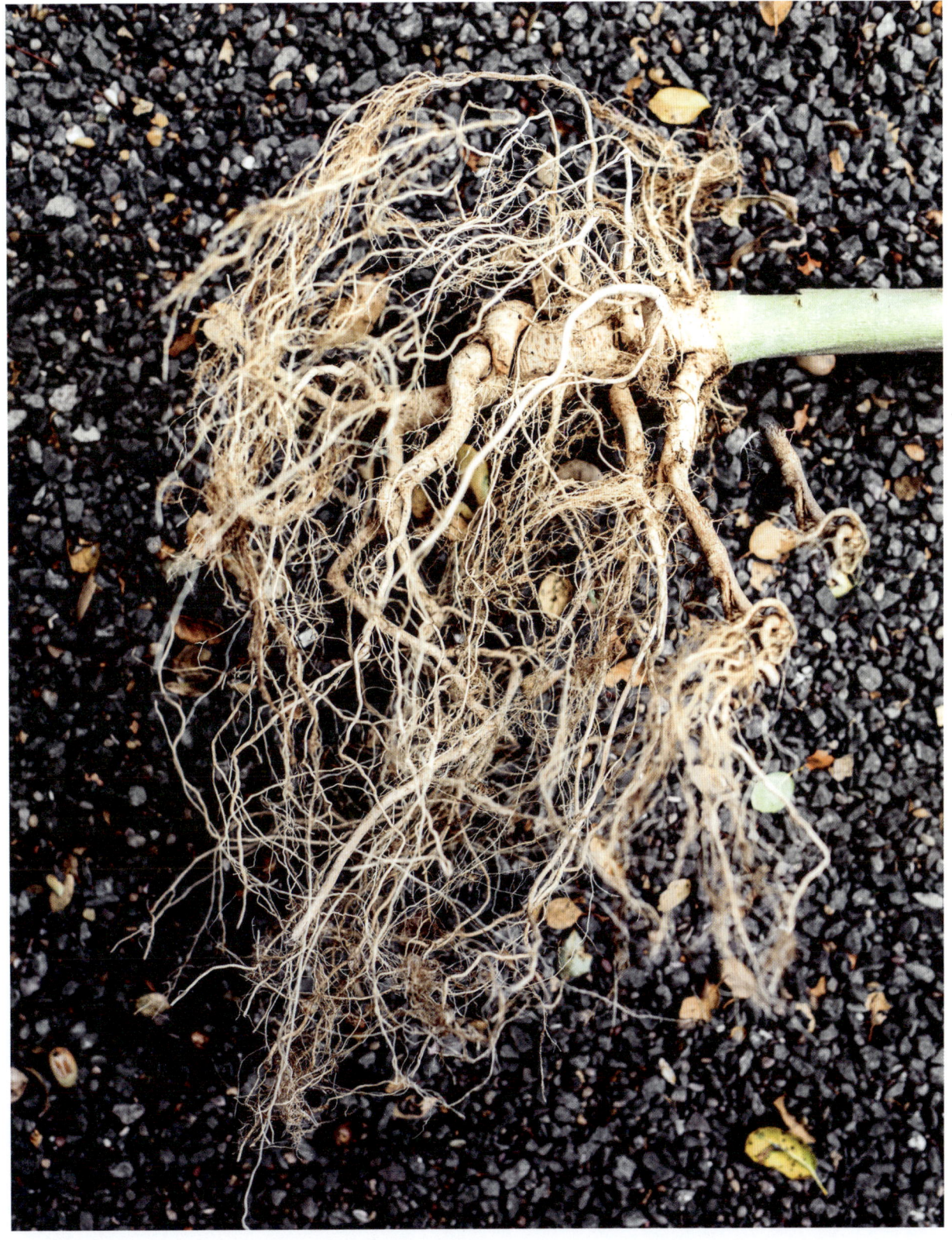

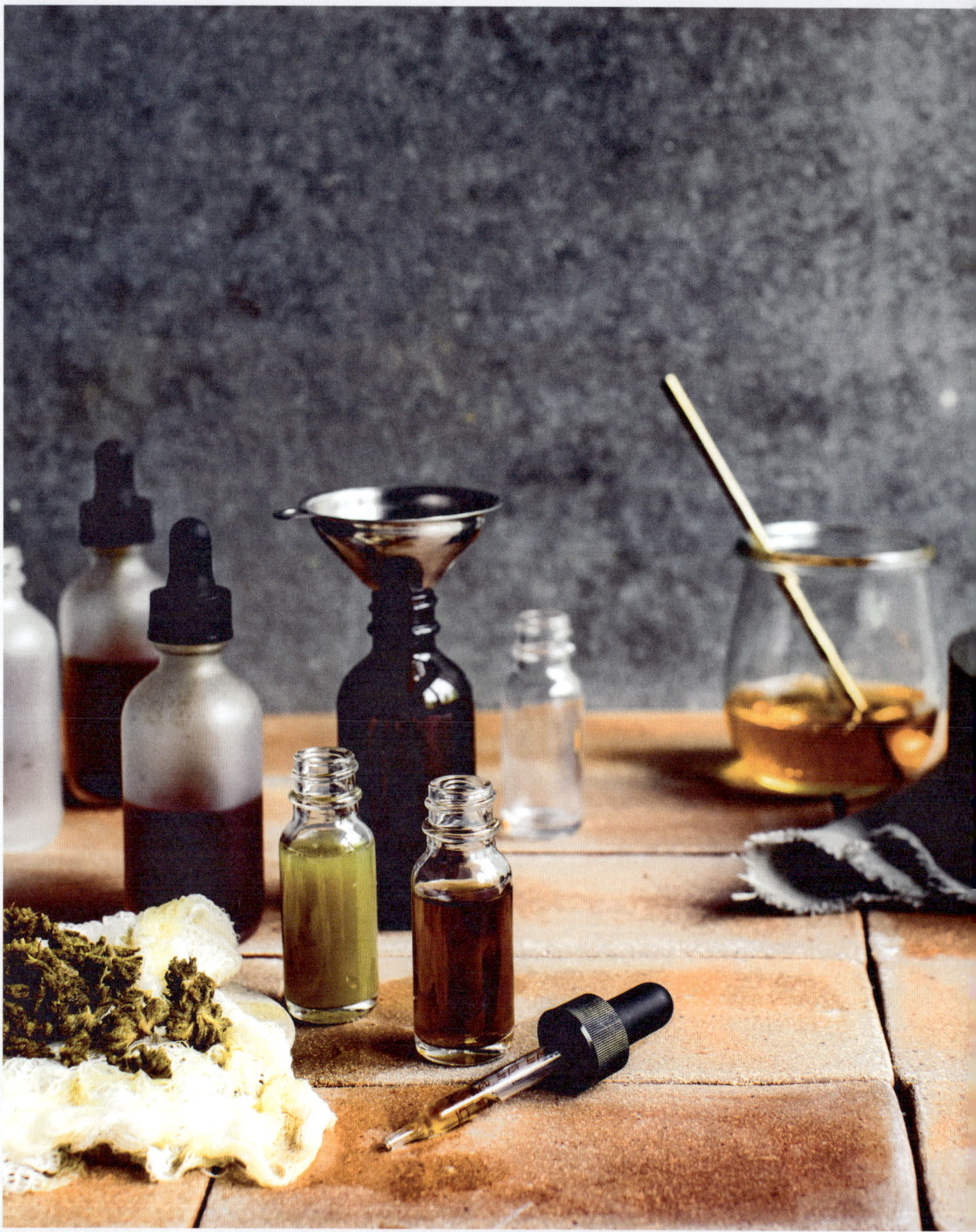

CHAPTER 8

Savoring Your Grow:

Tincture, Concentrate, Cannabutter, and Tisane with Key Recipes

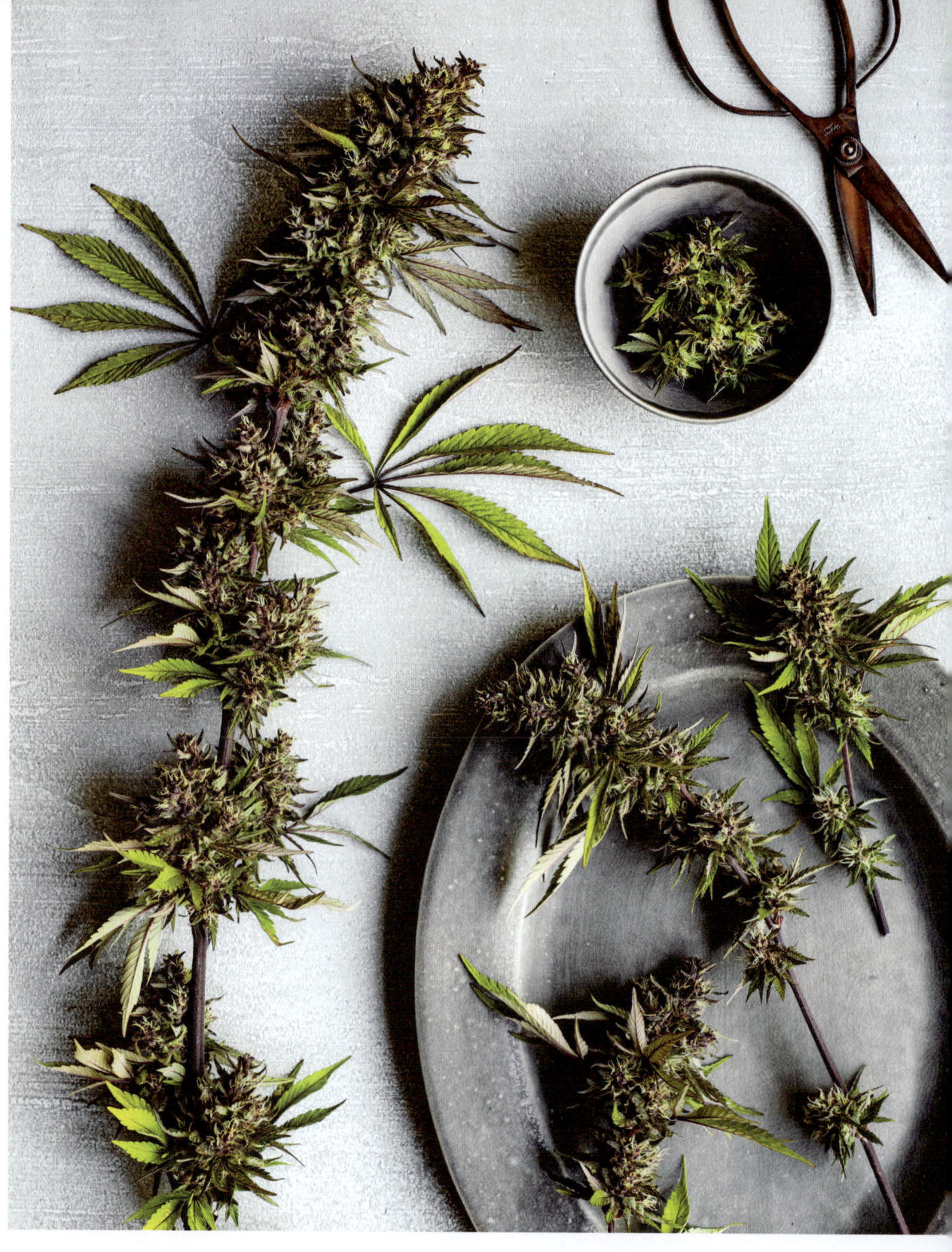

Now, if you wish, you can move into the kitchen with your grow. You can make your own edibles, tinctures, and topicals, using simple equipment and a few trustworthy recipes. If you've ever walked into a dispensary and wondered how you could make some of their products yourself—now you can. Do a little cost comparison, and you'll quickly realize how valuable your homegrown bud is. If you had a healthy crop, especially if you grew more than one full-size plant, you will likely have abundant weed available for use. As I discussed earlier, dried cannabis flower changes over time (see page 134), but properly stored dried and cured cannabis bud will remain potent and fresh for at least a year. Want to extend the life span of your grow tenfold? Make a tincture. Creating a tincture with your home-grown weed will "lock" the cannabinoids in place, and they will remain potent and fresh for years. I store my tinctures in the freezer, where they will stay strong and stable for a decade—maybe even longer. You have several options for kitchen craft with your grow—including beverages and edibles, both savory and sweet. Cannabinoids need to bind to either fat or alcohol—so all of my recipes will utilize one or the other. The exception to this is tisanes; here, terpenes rather than cannabinoids are the star, so no need for fat or alcohol to move cannabinoids into the hot water.

As the lifting of cannabis restrictions continues to grow and plant production increases, scientists are eagerly investigating the biochemistry of cannabis. They are rapidly gaining a new understanding of the many different cannabinoids in our modern cannabis strains and are learning more about THC and CBD, the two most abundant cannabinoids in weed. With this new information, they will able to predict with more accuracy what specific effects each cultivar will likely have on the user.

When you chose your cannabis plants, you likely considered what cannabinoids they express in their flowers (see pages 20–21). You may have leaned toward a high THC variety, a 1:1, or a strain with abundant CBD and little THC. No matter which strain you planted, you can fine-tune the impact of your weed on your body by knowing how to control the expression of cannabinoids in your creations and by understanding and managing proper dosing.

Decarboxylation

Contrary to much of the information you may have read, your cannabis is fully active and ready to enjoy whether or not you "decarboxylate" it—it's just that the cannabinoid profile will be different. Simply put, decarboxylation means *to remove a carboxyl group from a molecule*, and it's a common chemistry concept. While the word may be unfamiliar to some, the concept is pretty simple. The cannabinoids in raw cannabis begin in acid form (with the carboxyl group) in the bud and leaves. When you heat your bud, either by smoking raw flower or baking the bud in the oven, this carboxyl group moves off the cannabinoid molecule, creating a new cannabinoid. Most notably, THCa becomes THC, and CBDa becomes CBD. This is an important distinction, because THCa and THC impact your body very differently. THCa will not get you high, but THC will. CBDa and CBD are both effective but in different ways. Understanding this little bit of chemistry will allow you to feel confident that your cannabis creations will give you the health and mood impacts you want and fewer of the impacts you don't want. One of the decisions you'll need to make regarding your cannabis kitchen craft is whether or not to decarboxylate your bud before using it in recipes. If you want to maximize the THC in your tinctures, for example, you will need to fully decarboxylate the bud before using. If you're interested in managing inflammation with little psychotropic impact

THCa ➤ THC
(Δ9–tetrahydrocannabinol)

CBDa ➤ CBD
(Cannabidiol)

CBGa ➤ CBG
(Cannabigerol)

CBCa ➤ CBC
(Cannabichromene)

THC ➤ CBN

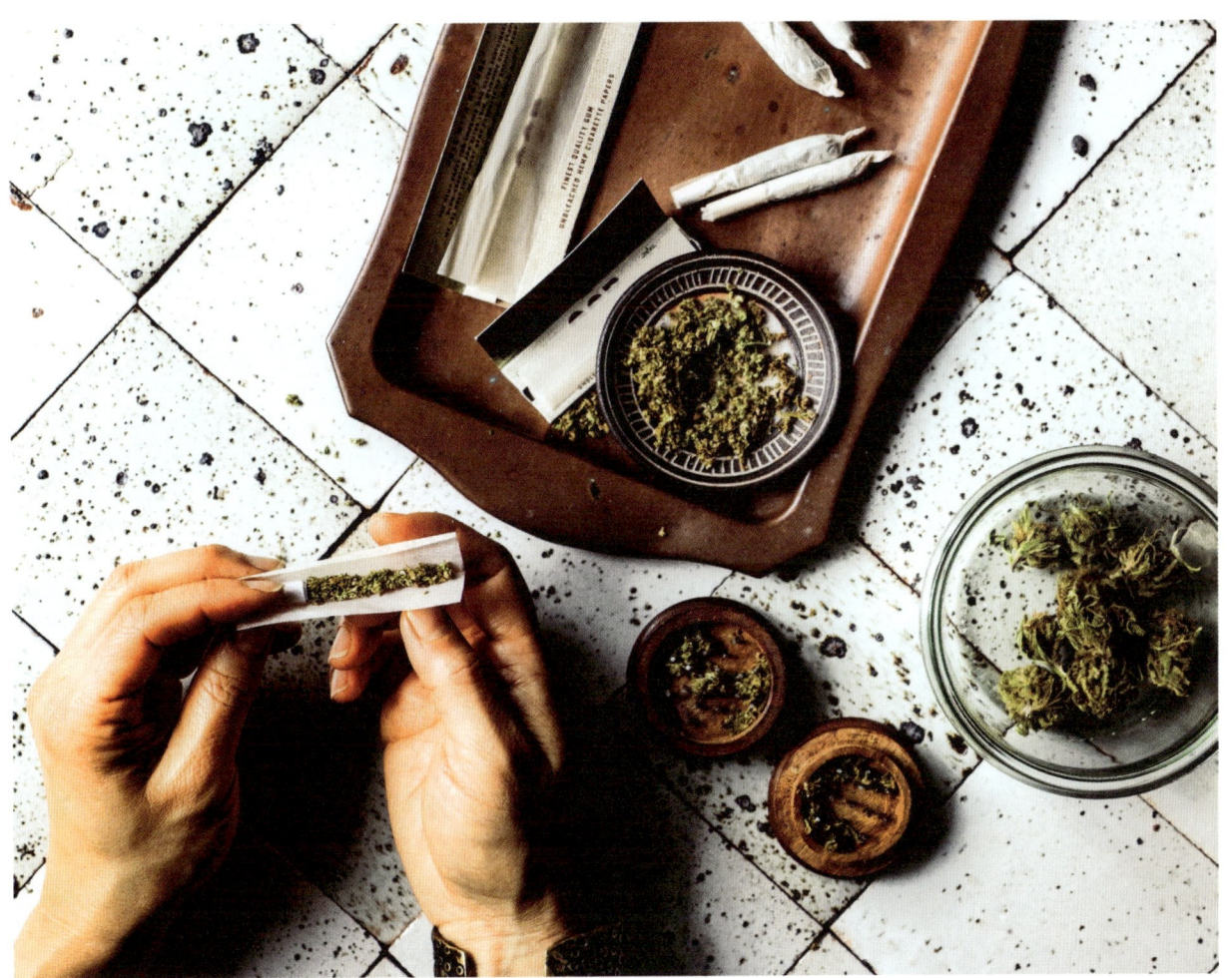

(that is, with no high), then use raw cannabis to retain the potent anti-inflammation impact of THCa and CBDa. *You* are in charge of your cannabis.

The Entourage Effect: Cannabinoids + Terpenes + You

Terpenes have a physiological as well as aesthetic effect and have a big impact on how cannabinoids act in your body; this is known as the entourage effect. Terpenes are what we smell when we brush our fingers over flower buds, and they are common in various plants. Lemon, pine, mango, lavender, cinnamon, and many other herbs, fruit, and spices smell good because of terpenes. You can also manipulate how "terpy" your cannabis creations are. In general, since terpenes are volatile, you will need to process your cannabis quickly using low temperatures to preserve the most terpenes. Freezing fresh cannabis bud and then making a tisane is an ideal way to maximize your terpenes (see page 172).

Potency and Dosing

One additional variable to keep in mind as you explore cannabis for your health concerns is potency and dosing. How much cannabis you consume, and how you consume it, makes a big impact on your experience. I offer a brief outline of consumption methods, with onset and duration, below. While vaping offers nearly the same impact as smoking, I do not advocate vaping, since there are too many unknown health risks in today's rapidly expanding product market, especially with those products found in the illicit market—yet another good reason to grow your own.

Cannabis Preparations, with Onset and Duration

CONSUMPTION METHOD	ONSET	DURATION	BEST USES	NOTES
Smoking	Immediately	30 minutes to 3 hours	Social settings; immediate relief	Avoid smoking to protect lung health
Tincture/ sublingual	10 to 15 minutes	30 minutes to several hours	Anytime you want fast relief	Discrete and good for accurate dosing
Edibles	1 to 3 hours	3 to several hours	When you desire a long duration effect	Modify potency in edibles by adjusting amount of infused ingredients
Topical	15 minutes	Several hours	Won't get you high; fights skin irritation	Ideal for localized body pain

Low and Slow: How to Dose Your Weed for Best Effect

Potency matters—usually! Knowing the onset and duration of your preparations is important to help you know how to get what you want from your weed. One of the biggest mistakes that newbies make is starting with an edible. Here's an all too common story that I've heard many times from folks who attend my Cannabis 101 education events. The story goes something like this: "My friend gave me some cannabis-infused brownie. I took a bite but didn't feel anything, so I ate some more—and still—nothing. Then I ate the whole thing, and after another hour, I felt weird, and dizzy, and then got really stoned, threw up, and went to bed." What a way to try cannabis for the first time. I offer the table opposite to help guide you, so you will know what to expect from your cannabis preparations.

Edibles. For edibles, there are two reasons to know the potency, especially of THC: its slow onset and the large variability with metabolism. Because edibles pass through the digestive system before hitting the bloodstream and then the endocannabinoid system (ECS), there are a number of significant variables that influence how quickly and for how long THC acts on the body. For example, if you eat the edible on an empty stomach, you'll digest it faster than if you had it at the end of a big, heavy meal. If your edible is fat based, it will affect you differently than if it's an alcohol-based edible. Additionally, as the THC passes through the liver, it is first converted to a different, more potent form of THC that creates a stronger impression of euphoria, or psychedelic experience, than the same amount of THC consumed in a different way. Edibles have a long duration, too, so once you eat some, you're going to be impacted for several hours. Knowing this is helpful. Edibles can be the best way to have a long duration effect, which is great for those times when you want to be pain-free or extra-relaxed for several hours.

Smokable flower and sublingual tinctures. The potency of smokable flower and sublingual tinctures matters, but it is easily discernible by the imbiber because of the fast onset of the effect. Smoking has the fastest onset, usually happening within minutes of consumption, and offers the quickest duration. Sublinguals are nearly as fast an onset with a somewhat longer duration. While it's a nice to have an estimate of the potency of your flower or tincture preparation, it's not essential. You'll know quickly enough how to dose with these applications.

Topicals. The one preparation where potency is not a concern is with topicals. The reason is that the skin is the body's barrier to the outside world and is thus resistant to allowing substances to move very readily from the skin's surface to the bloodstream. This doesn't mean that the cannabinoids and terpenes aren't effective in topical applications—quite the contrary. They are powerfully active but offer shallow penetration into the area surrounding the application of the topical salve or oil. This is great news for those who want excellent pain relief for joints and muscles or to treat minor skin infections and inflammation without psychoactivity. I make very concentrated salves using a small kitchen device called the Source Turbo (see Sources, page 178). I find that my homemade salves work better than any commercial preparations I've tried, and I think it's because they are jam-packed with cannabinoids (see page 159).

RECIPES

Making simple, effective, and delicious creations with home-grown cannabis is one my great joys in life. Here I share key techniques for harnessing the healing agents in your bud and moving them into concentrate, tincture, and fat. These three key infused ingredients are then used in original recipes to craft your own salve, edible treats, and soothing elixir. Cannabis tisane combinations are offered to make delicious use of dried leaves. These recipes are simple to make and use common kitchen equipment. I rely on a digital kitchen scale for most of my baking, finding it helpful for accurate measurement. The one unusual piece of equipment I use is a tabletop extractor (see above), important for making highly concentrated salve.

How to Decarboxylate Your Dried Bud

Decarboxylation is the process of converting THCa to THC, and CBDa to CBD in your dried cannabis bud. It is an important step for managing the cannabinoid profile in your recipes. "Decarbing" weed is smelly, so use proper ventilation while baking and cooling.

Preheat the oven to 240°F. Line a rimmed baking sheet with parchment paper.

Scatter the bud evenly on the prepared baking sheet and place the pan on the middle rack of the oven. Bake for 25 minutes, then remove the pan from the oven. The green bud will emerge from the oven a little duller in color but should not be too toasty looking. The fragrance will be strong, with a slightly roasted character. Carefully transfer the parchment from the hot baking sheet onto a heatproof surface or wire rack, then place on a draft-free counter. Allow to cool for 10 minutes, then use straightaway in recipes or store airtight in a cool, dark place until ready to use.

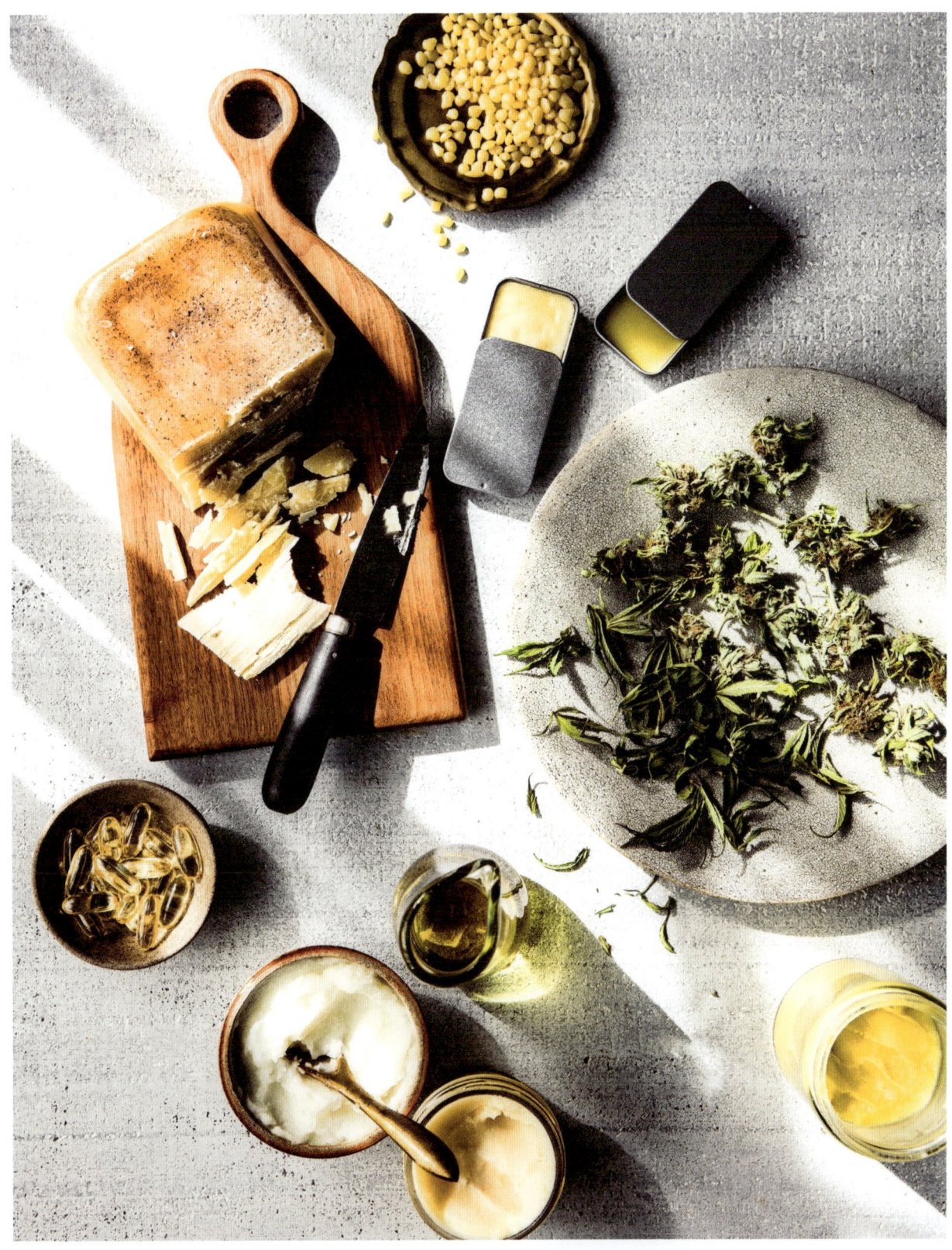

Cannabis Tincture

MAKES ABOUT
1¼ CUPS

This is a concentrated high-alcohol cannabis tincture. Using a neutral high-alcohol spirit allows for the best transfer of cannabinoids into the tincture. Each state has different alcohol proof limits—get the highest proof you can find. Chilling the alcohol before using it minimizes the transfer of strong-flavored fats and chlorophyll from bud to tincture, allowing for a rich, smooth flavor. While I specify bud in the following recipe, you may also use sugar leaves to make high-quality tinctures. Tincture is my favorite way to consume cannabis, as it is easy to accurately dose and has a fast onset when taken sublingually. This tincture is also wonderful for using in cocktails and for making water-based edibles, including Vanilla Bean–Infused Gummies (page 151) and Fresh Satsuma–Infused Gummies (page 152).

Notes on fine-tuning cannabinoids in your tincture:

> For THC/CBD in your tincture, decarboxylate your dried bud before making the tincture (see page 144).

> For THCa/CBDa in your tincture, use raw dried bud.

> For extra terpene flavor, make a tincture with fresh bud, either straight from the plant or frozen at harvest.

35g to 40g dried cannabis bud, chopped	1½ cups very cold highest-potency neutral grain alcohol (chill in the freezer for 2 hours prior to use)

To extract the bud: Pack the bud pieces into a widemouthed glass container with a lid. Pour the alcohol onto the bud, leaving a small headspace at the top of the jar. Cover and place the jar in the freezer. Give the mixture

CONTINUED

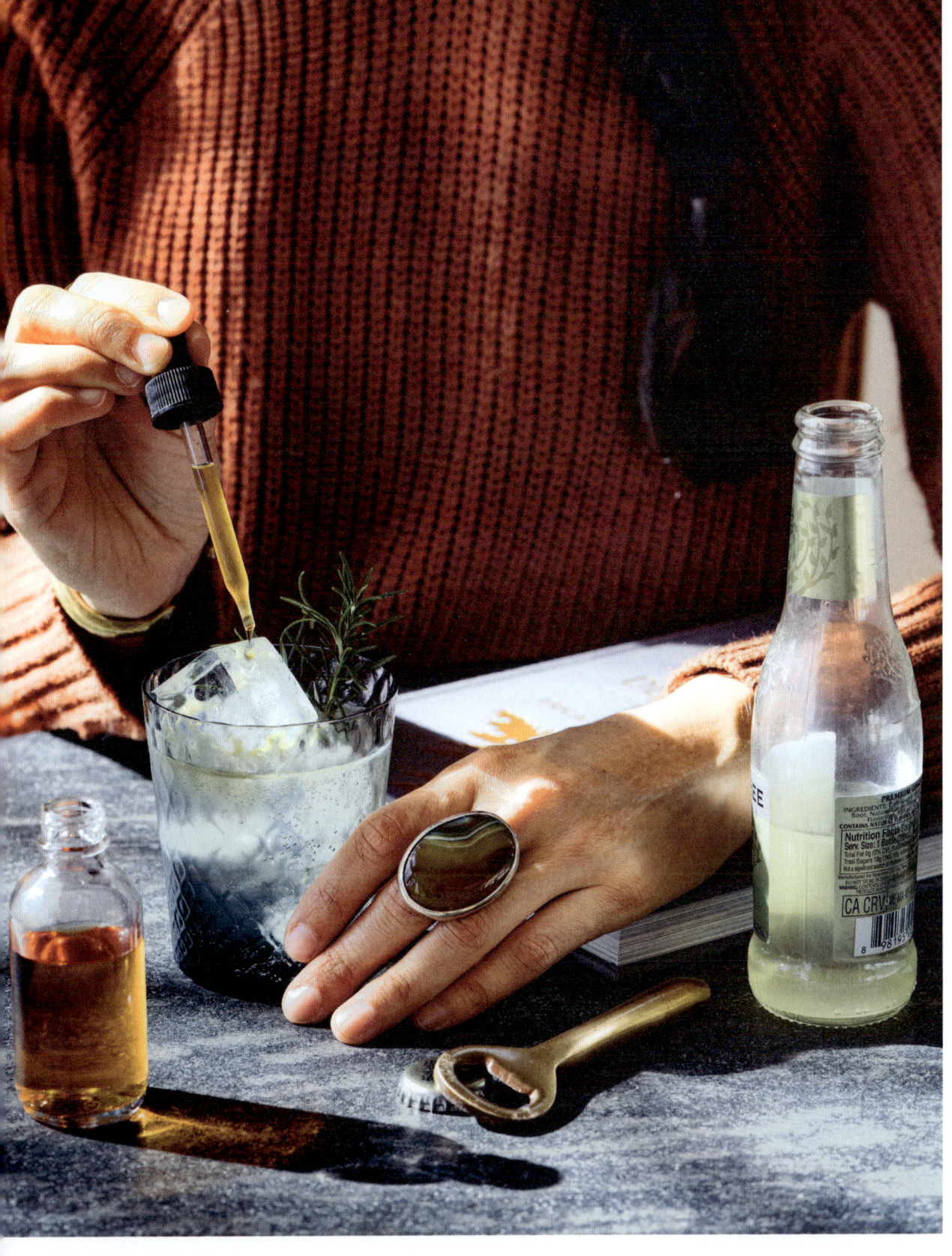

a gentle swirl every couple of hours. The mixture should remain in the freezer for 3 to 5 days to achieve full extraction.

To strain and store: Line a strainer with several layers of cheesecloth or a nutmilk bag and place the strainer over a clean glass bowl or a measuring cup big enough to hold the liquid. Pour the cannabis-alcohol mixture into the strainer.

After most of the liquid has passed through, gather up the corners of the cheesecloth and twist them together to push the cannabis bud into the belly of the fabric. Grasp the gathered cloth and squeeze firmly to release as much liquid as possible.

For greater final tincture clarity, filter the tincture again by pouring the tincture through a coffee filter, using a cone drip holder.

Decant the tincture into small dark-colored glass bottles. Cap with a rubber dropper lid. For longer-term storage, close with a nonrubber cap. Stored in airtight glass containers in the freezer, this tincture will remain potent for a decade or more. Be sure to label with the date, cultivar, and whether or not you decarbed your bud.

BONUS: If you'd like to enjoy a cannabis-infused soak, place the spent bud in a clean piece of cheesecloth and gather the cheesecloth into a ball around the bud, securing it with cotton string. Steep this in a hot bath, enjoying the herbal smell as it wafts out of the water. Compost the spent cannabis bud.

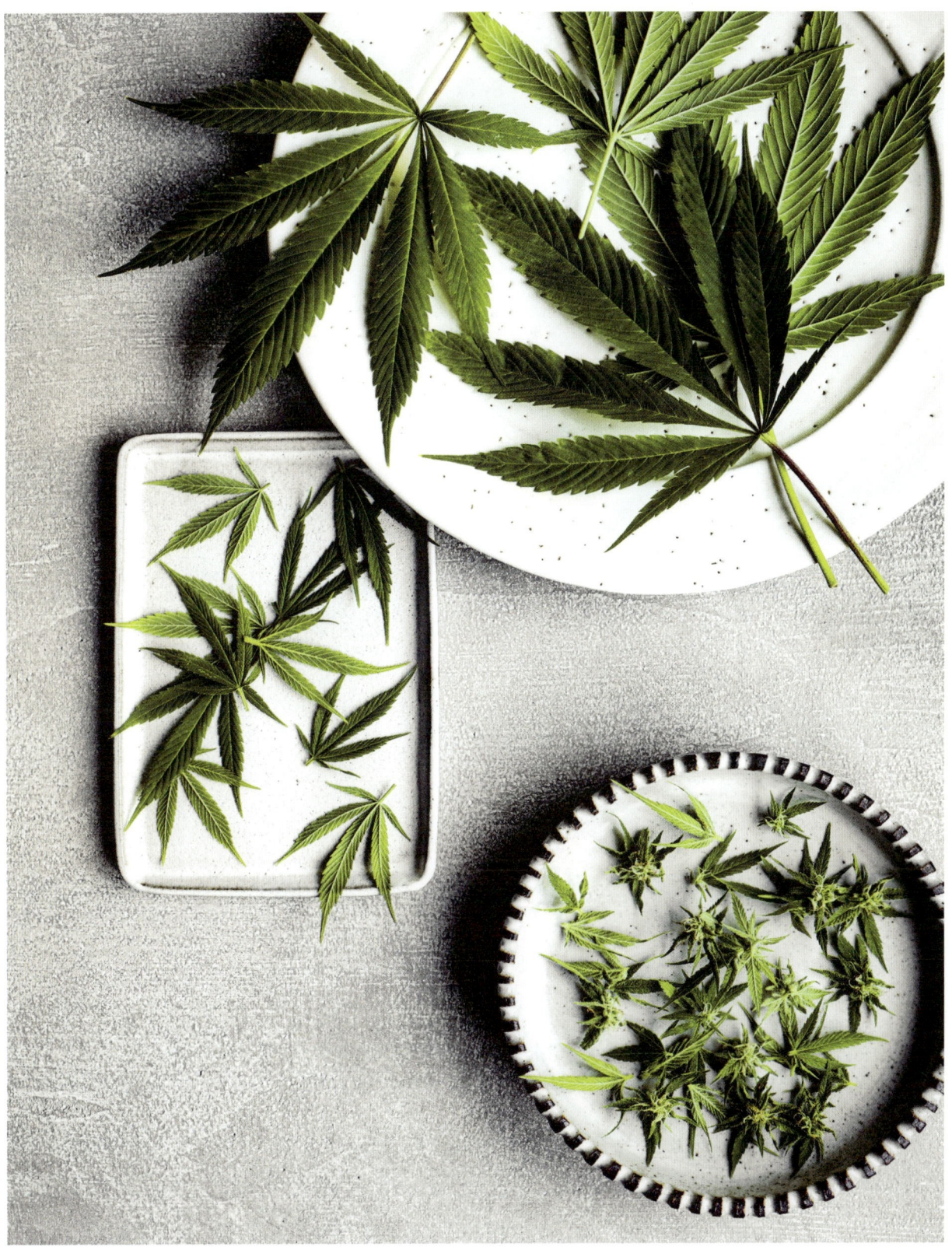

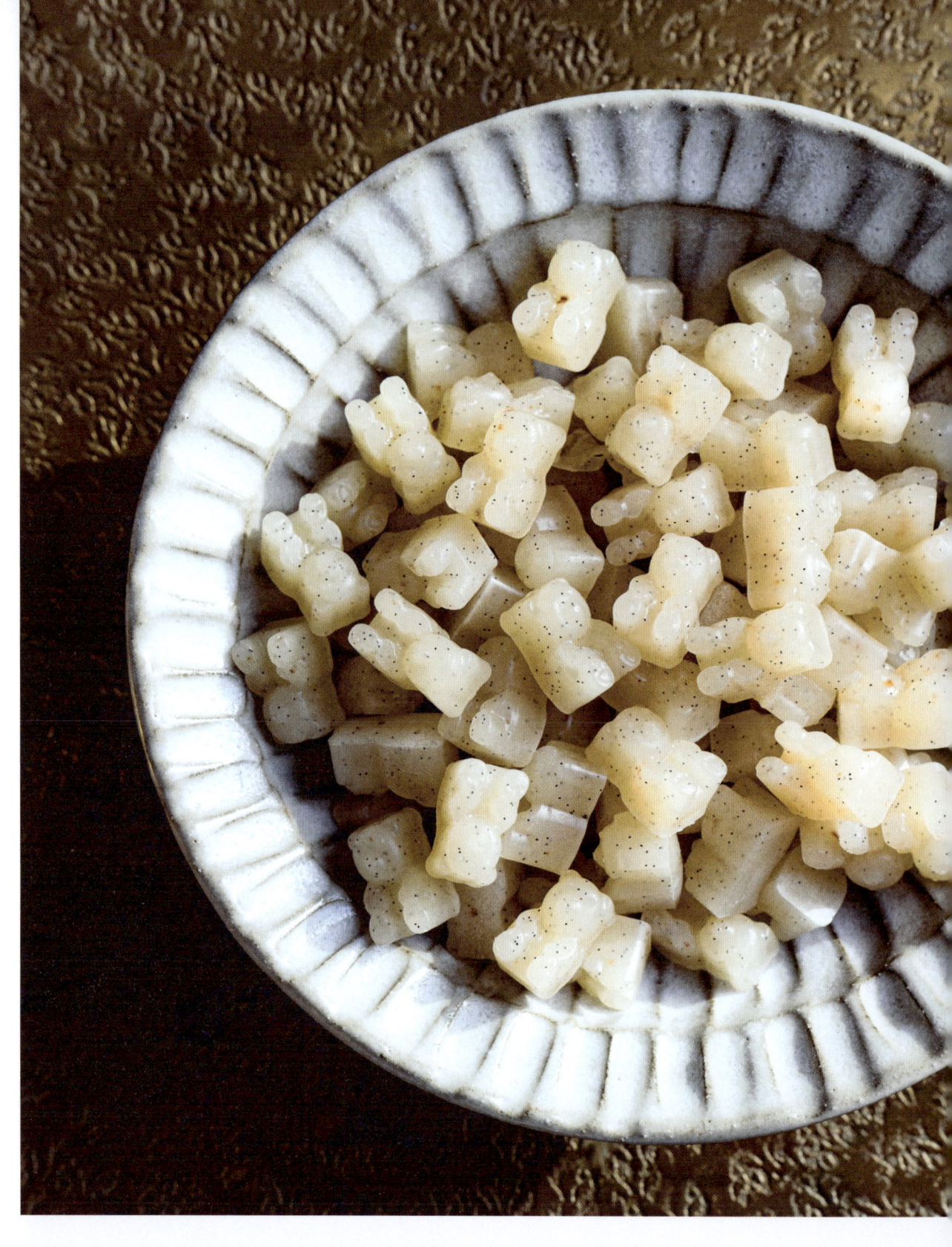

Vanilla Bean–Infused Gummies

Infused gummies are the perfect vehicle for low-dose cannabis consumption. You will first need to make the cannabis tincture. The cannabinoid profile for these gummies will naturally be the same as in your tincture, with three gummy bears equivalent to one dropperful (⅛ teaspoon) of tincture. If you don't have access to a silicone mold, you may use an 8 by 8-inch baking pan instead. Allow the mixture to solidfy, then cut the gelled mixture into small ¾-inch squares.

5 tablespoons full fat, unsweetened coconut milk

1 tablespoon Cannabis Tincture (page 146)

5 tablespoons sugar

1 teaspoon vanilla extract

½ vanilla bean, split, seeds scraped and reserved

Dash of salt, preferably fine-grain

4 teaspoons unflavored gelatin

In a 1-pint glass measuring cup, combine the coconut milk, tincture, sugar, vanilla extract and seeds, salt, and gelatin. Allow the mixture to rest at room temperature for 3 minutes to bloom the gelatin.

Heat the mixture in the microwave on high for 45 seconds. Stir, then heat on high for an additional 15 seconds. Stir again and pour into silicone gummy bear molds. Cool before removing from the molds, then store in an airtight container in the fridge for up to a month or in the freezer for up to a year.

Fresh Satsuma–Infused Gummies

MAKES ABOUT 65 GUMMIES

Sweet, tart Satsuma mandarins offer delicious bright flavor to these juicy gummies. Any good quality citrus will work in this recipe. If you use lemon or lime instead of Satsuma, substitute water for half of the juice for best flavor balance.

Finely grated zest of 1 Satsuma mandarin (about ½ teaspoon)

5 tablespoons fresh squeezed Satsuma mandarin juice

5 tablespoons granulated sugar

1 tablespoon Cannabis Tincture (page 146)

4 teaspoons unflavored gelatin

In a 1-pint glass measuring cup, mix the mandarin zest, mandarin juice, sugar, tincture, and gelatin. Allow to rest at room temperature for 3 minutes to bloom the gelatin.

Heat the mixture in the microwave on high for 45 seconds. Stir well, then heat the mixture on high for an additional 15 seconds if needed. Stir again, then pour into silicone molds. Cool before removing from the molds, then store in an airtight container in the fridge for up to a month or in the freezer for up to a year.

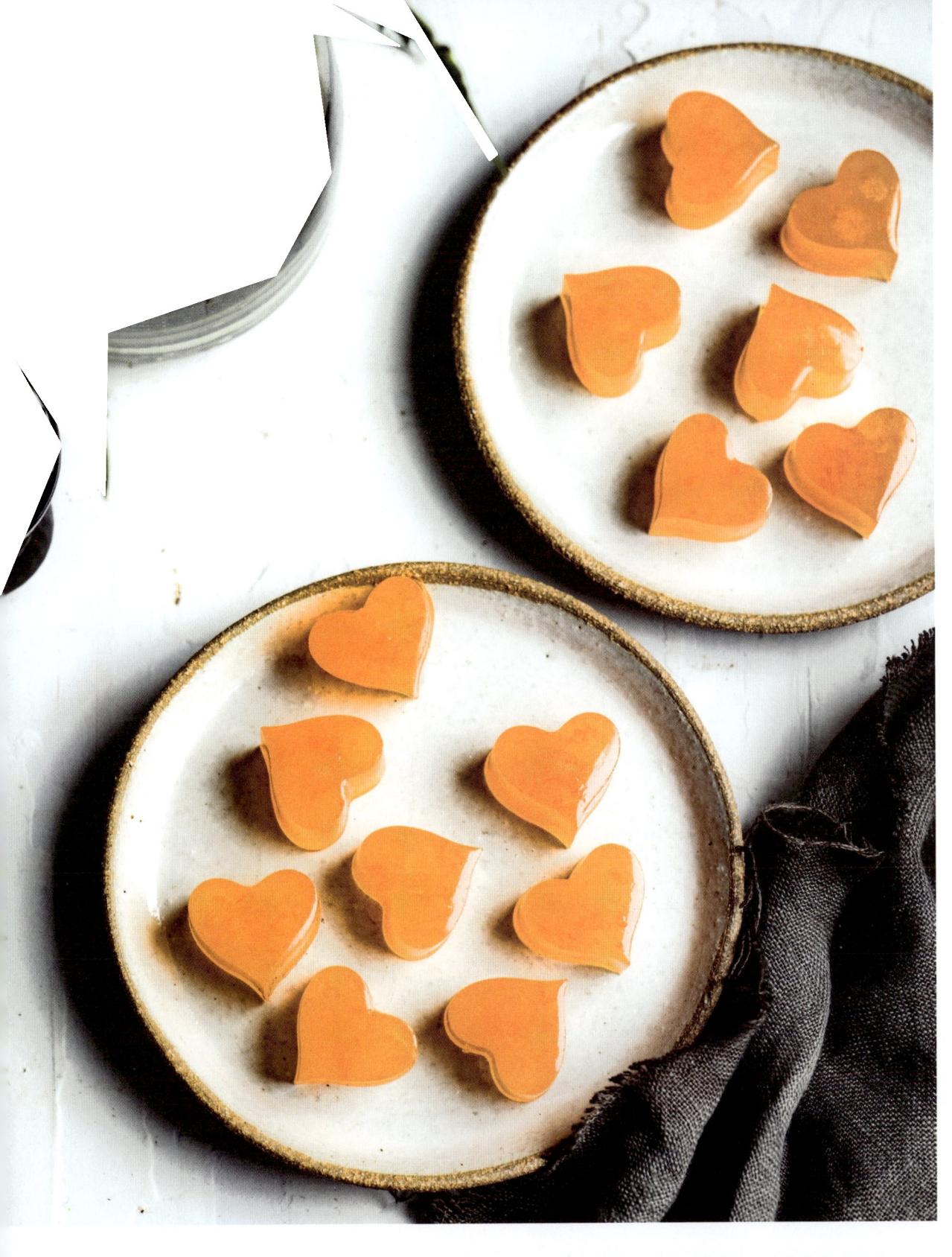

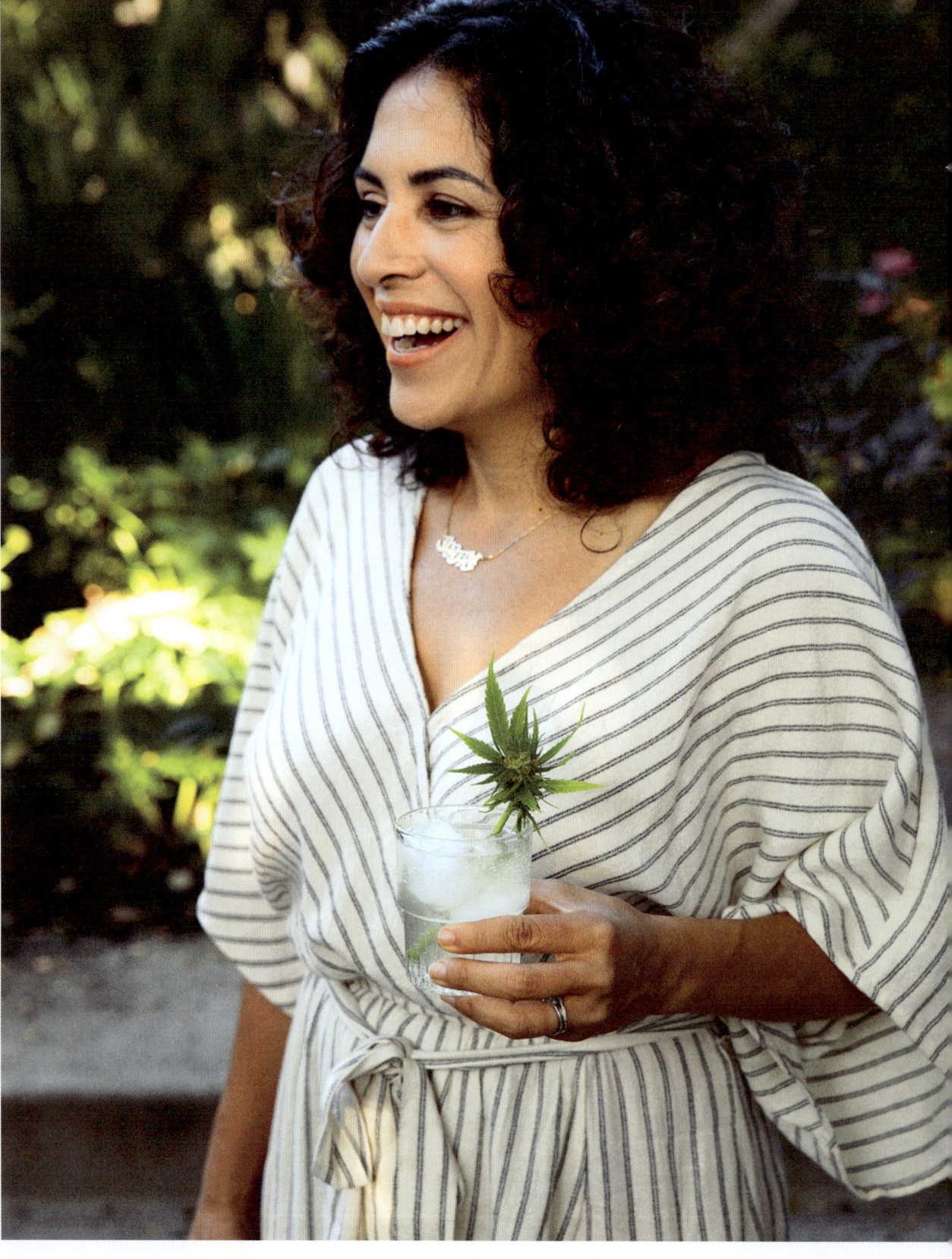

Canna-Ginger Refresher

SERVES 1

My favorite cannabis mocktail ever! I particularly love to enjoy this post workout. I make raw tinctures that I use generously in this drink—the THCa and CBDa are excellent anti-inflammatory agents and help me recover from exercise. This beverage is helpful for indigestion as well. But really? I love it because it's so delicious. The effects are similar to taking some tincture but with slower onset. You may use any amount of tincture in this recipe, depending on how you respond to your particular batch. For the ginger beer, my favorite brand is Fever-Tree.

7 ounces cold ginger beer

¼ teaspoon Cannabis Tincture (page 146) or to taste

Lime wedge

Cannabis leaf, rosemary sprig, or thyme sprig for garnish

Combine the ginger beer and the tincture in a cold pint glass. Squeeze the lime wedge into the mixture, add ice, garnish with a cannabis leaf, and enjoy.

Cannabis Concentrate

A cannabis concentrate is an oily liquid composed almost entirely of the cannabinoids and terpene-rich resins made by the cannabis plant. This dark green/black concentrate is loaded with cannabinoids to use in topicals or consumed in tiny quantities for a powerful impact. To make it, I use a Source Turbo extractor (see Sources, page 178), which is a tabletop device that helps to preserve the integrity of the concentrate by keeping the temperature at or below 100°F, while evaporating and recovering ethanol with vacuum pressures. I use only 100 percent pure food-grade ethanol. If you are unable to find food-grade ethanol, you may substitute a high-proof neutral spirit such as Everclear. Do *not* use isopropyl alcohol or denatured alcohol for this recipe; those are not food-grade products.

50g dried decarboxylated cannabis bud (see page 144), chopped

1 pint (2 cups) food-grade 100% (200 proof) ethanol

Lightly pack the cannabis in a widemouthed 1-quart glass container with a lid. Pour the ethanol over the cannabis and close the container. Allow the cannabis/ethanol mixture to rest for an hour. Gently agitate the container every 10 minutes to facilitate the movement of the cannabinoids into the ethanol.

Using several layers of cheesecloth or a nutmilk bag, strain the cannabis from the liquid into a glass measuring cup big enough to hold the liquid.

Strain the liquid again through a coffee filter, using a cone drip holder, for optimal clarity of the final concentrate.

Follow the extractor manufacturer's instructions to evaporate off the ethanol, reserving it for a future extraction.

Store the concentrate in an airtight glass container in the freezer for up to 2 years for best potency.

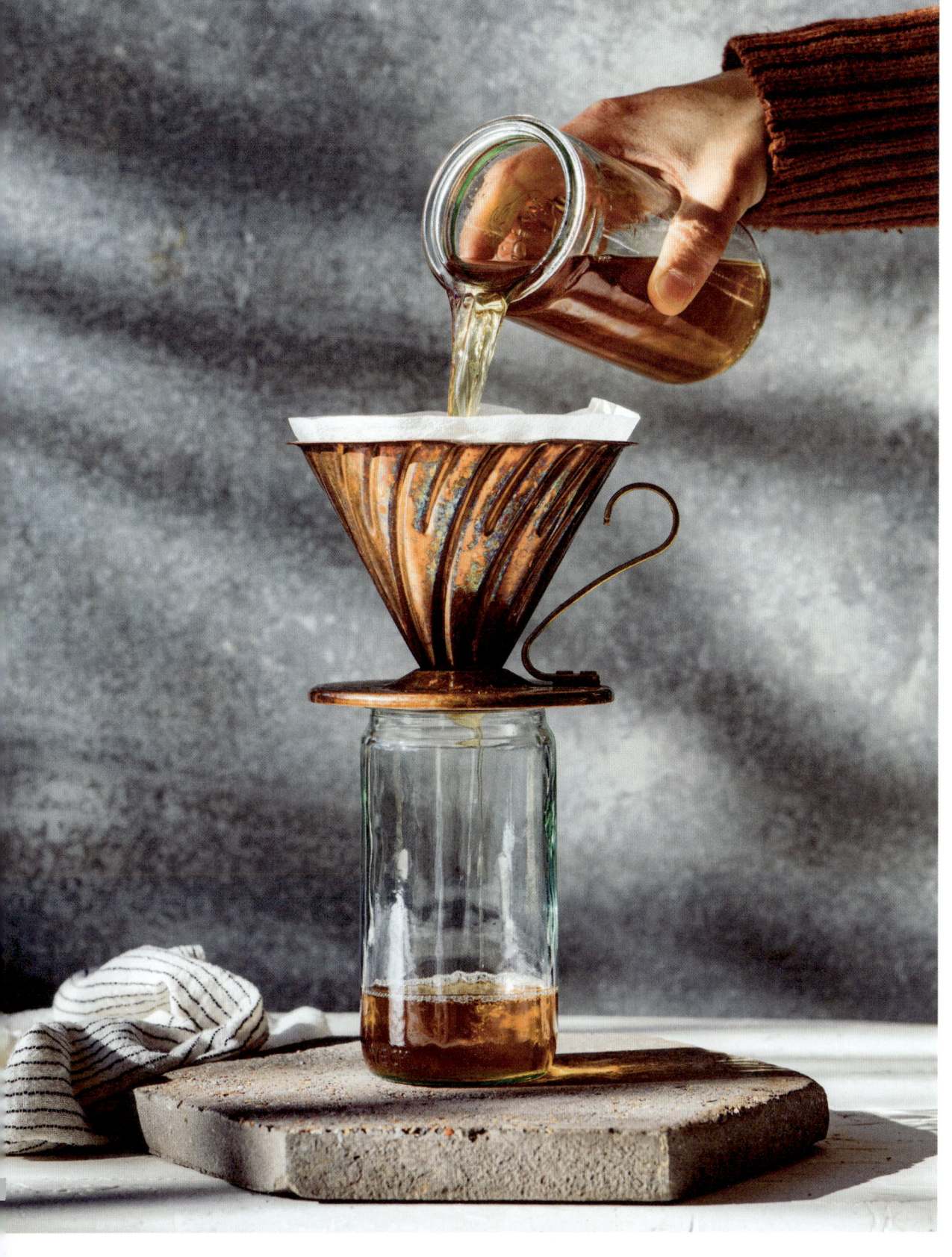

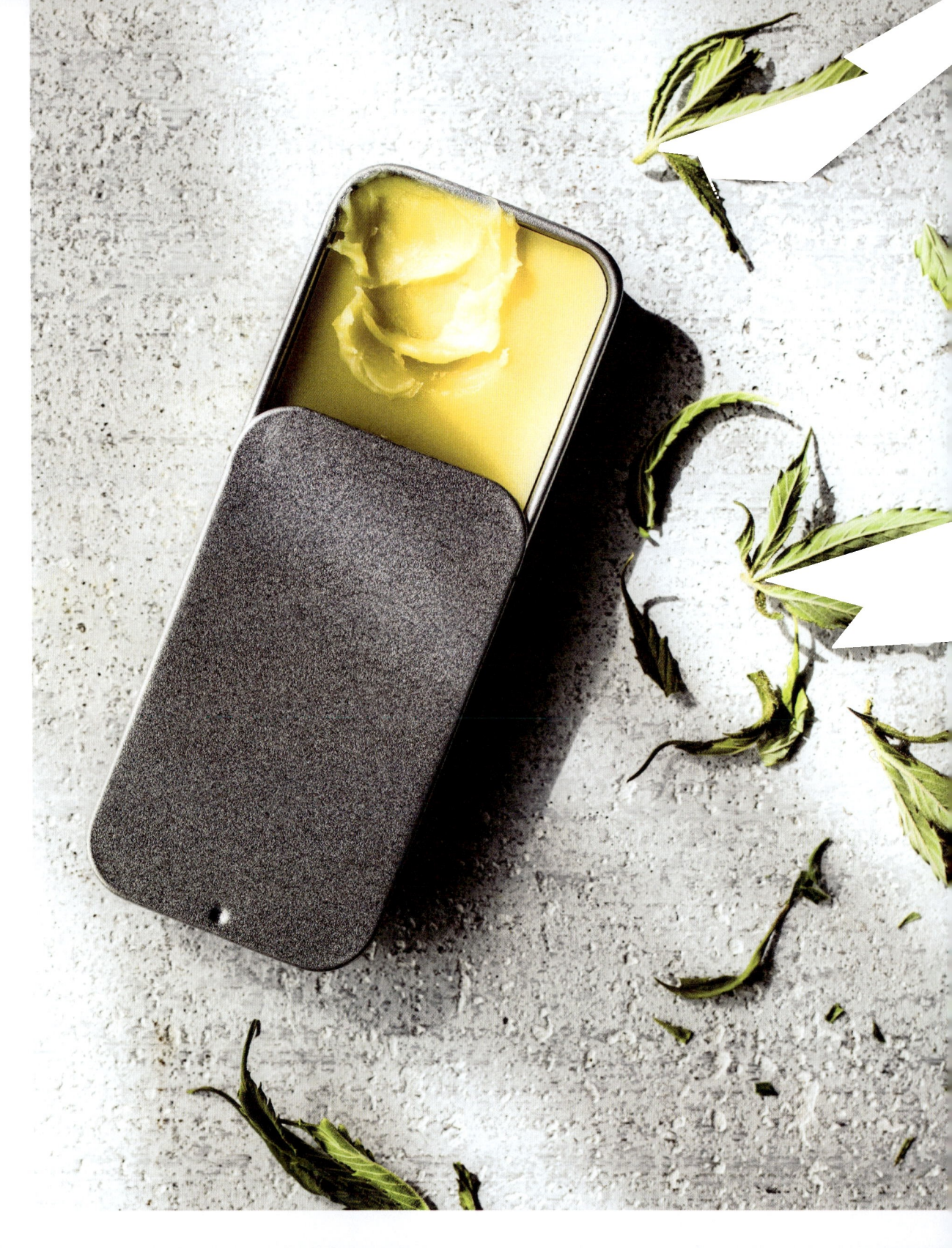

Cannabis Salve

MAKES 1½ CUPS

This silky-smooth salve made with cannabis concentrate works well to soothe aching muscles and joints. Non-intoxicating and safe for all skin types, it's an excellent balm for pain, inflammation, and for calming skin itchiness and irritations. I use refined virgin coconut oil to keep the coconut fragrance light. You may add essential oil if you enjoy scented salve.

⅔ cup (150g) shea butter

⅔ cup (150g) coconut oil

42g beeswax (45g for hot climates)

6 vitamin E capsules (180mg/capsule)

2 tablespoons Cannabis Concentrate (page 156)

12 drops essential oil (optional)

Fill a medium saucepan with 1 to 2 inches water and heat until simmering.

While the water is heating, combine the shea butter, coconut oil, and beeswax in a 1-quart glass or metal pitcher.

Place the pitcher in the simmering water, making sure that no water gets into the salve mixture, and stir until just melted. You will notice that the beeswax takes the longest to melt. Remove the pitcher from the heat.

Pierce the vitamin E capsules and squeeze the contents into the oil/cannabis mixture; do not add the vitamin E capsule casings. Add the cannabis concentrate and essential oil (if using) and stir the mixture to combine.

Quickly pour the liquid into small widemouthed glass or metal containers with lids. If the mixture begins to solidify before you've finished pouring it into the containers, reheat it over the simmering water.

You may find that the salve gets grainy after several months. This will not affect the quality of the salve, but if you prefer a smooth texture you may gently heat the salve over a hot water bath until it remelts. Let cool. The salve will return to its original velvety texture. Store in a cool dark spot for up to 2 years.

Cannabutter or Cannaoil

**MAKES ABOUT
1 POUND**

Cannabutter is the foundation of many delicious cannabis-infused foods. The cannabinoids in bud dissolve easily into the fat in butter or oil. Three recipes following this one offer a few ways to enjoy your cannabutter. Let the Cannabis Cheesy Goldfish Crackers (page 165), Infused Chocolate Shell (page 168), and Infused Chocolate Sauce (page 171) be starting points for your culinary cannabis fun.

The amount of cannabis bud you use here will determine the potency of the finished product. Because it is 100 percent fat, coconut oil offers slightly higher extraction of cannabinoids than butter. Most recipes are designed for a ratio of 16 ounces of fat to 1 ounce (28g) of cannabis, but you are free to alter the potency by increasing or decreasing the amount of dried cannabis in this recipe. To store, it's best to use a glass or metal container to block the transfer of odor to the other contents of your fridge.

1 pound unsalted butter
or coconut oil

20g to 40g packed dried
decarboxylated cannabis bud
(see page 144)

SLOW COOKER METHOD: Heat the slow cooker on high for 5 minutes, then turn to low. Add the butter or coconut oil and allow it to melt. Proceed to next step, Adding the Bud.

WATER BATH METHOD: Add 2 inches of water to a medium saucepan. Heat until the water is simmering. Place the butter or coconut oil into a medium glass or metal bowl that will fit over the pan without allowing the simmering water to touch or enter. Set the bowl over the simmering water to melt the butter or coconut oil.

CONTINUED

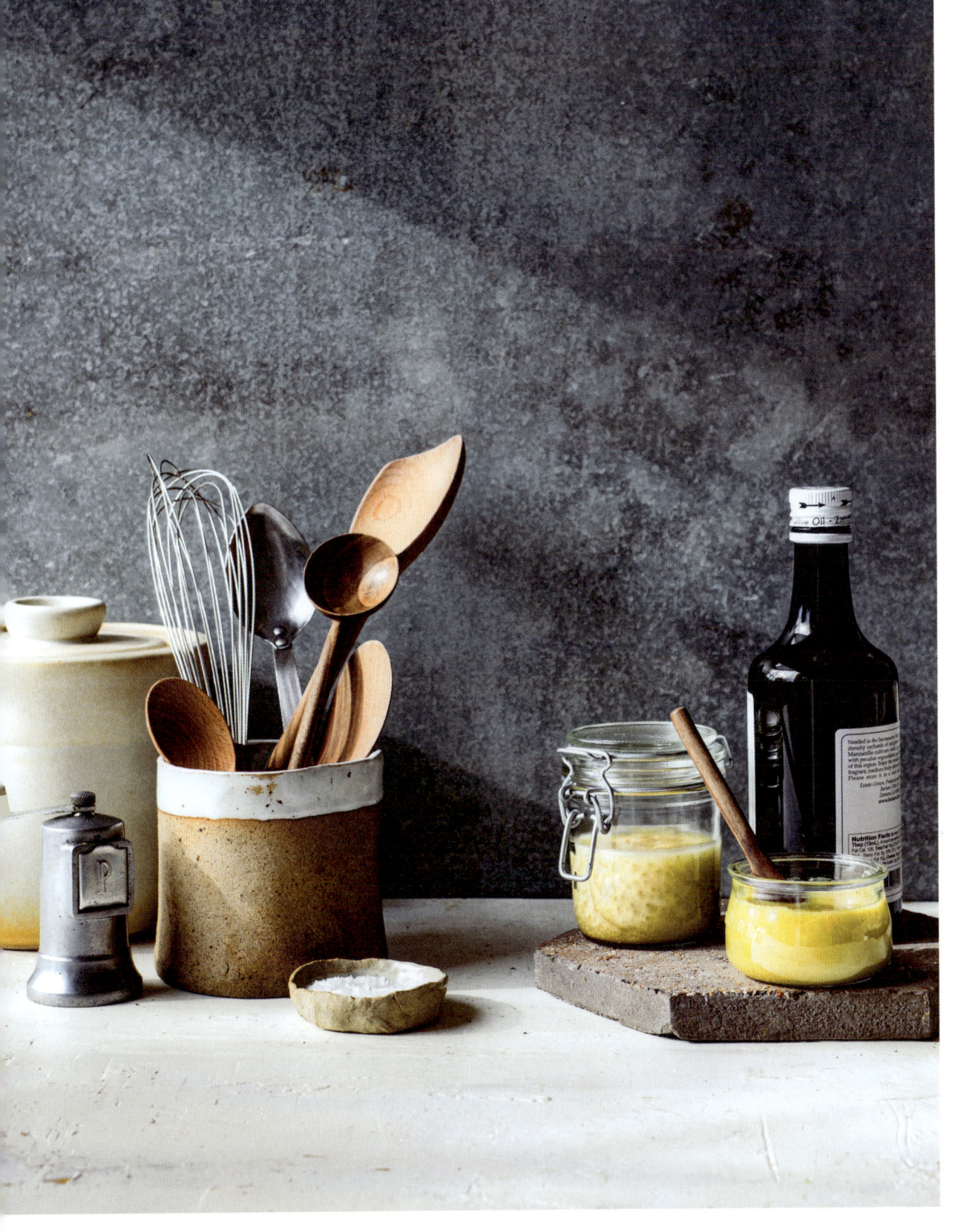

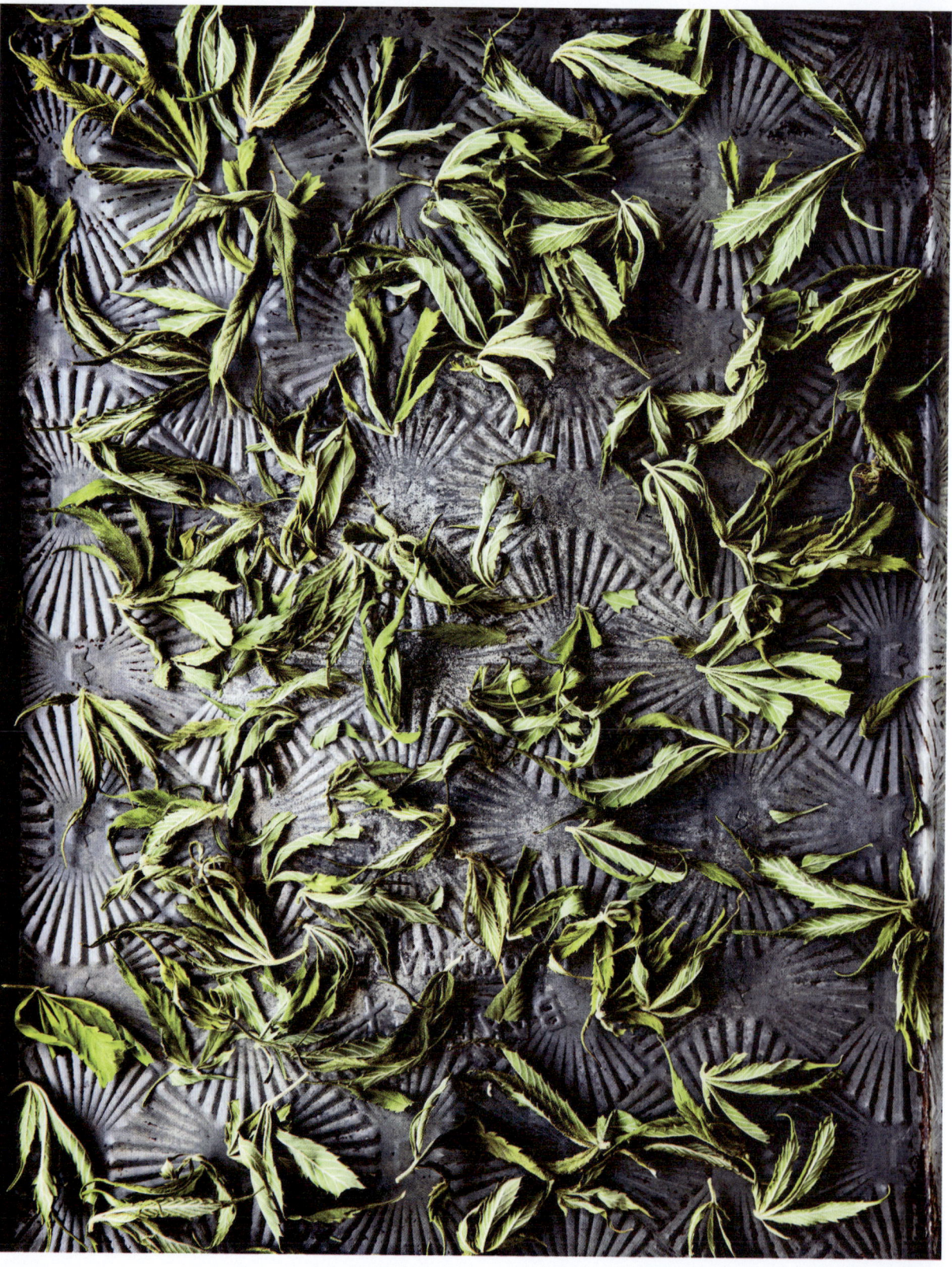

ADDING THE BUD: While the butter or coconut oil is melting, chop your bud into ¼- to ½-inch pieces to compact the volume of the bud and to increase contact with the fat. No need to grind the bud: the resins are on the bud surface, not inside the cell walls.

When the butter or coconut oil is melted, add the bud. Allow the cannabis/fat mixture to cook for 1 hour at a low temperature. Check the water level in the pan midway through the infusion time, adding more water to the pan if it gets lower than ½ inch, if using the water bath method.

STRAIN AND STORE: Line a strainer with several layers of cheesecloth or a nutmilk bag and place the strainer over a glass bowl or measuring cup big enough to hold the infused butter. Pour the mixture into the strainer, then discard the solids.

Store the cannabutter or cannaoil in an airtight container in the fridge for up to 1 month or for 6 months in the freezer. Cannaoil has a longer shelf life than cannabutter.

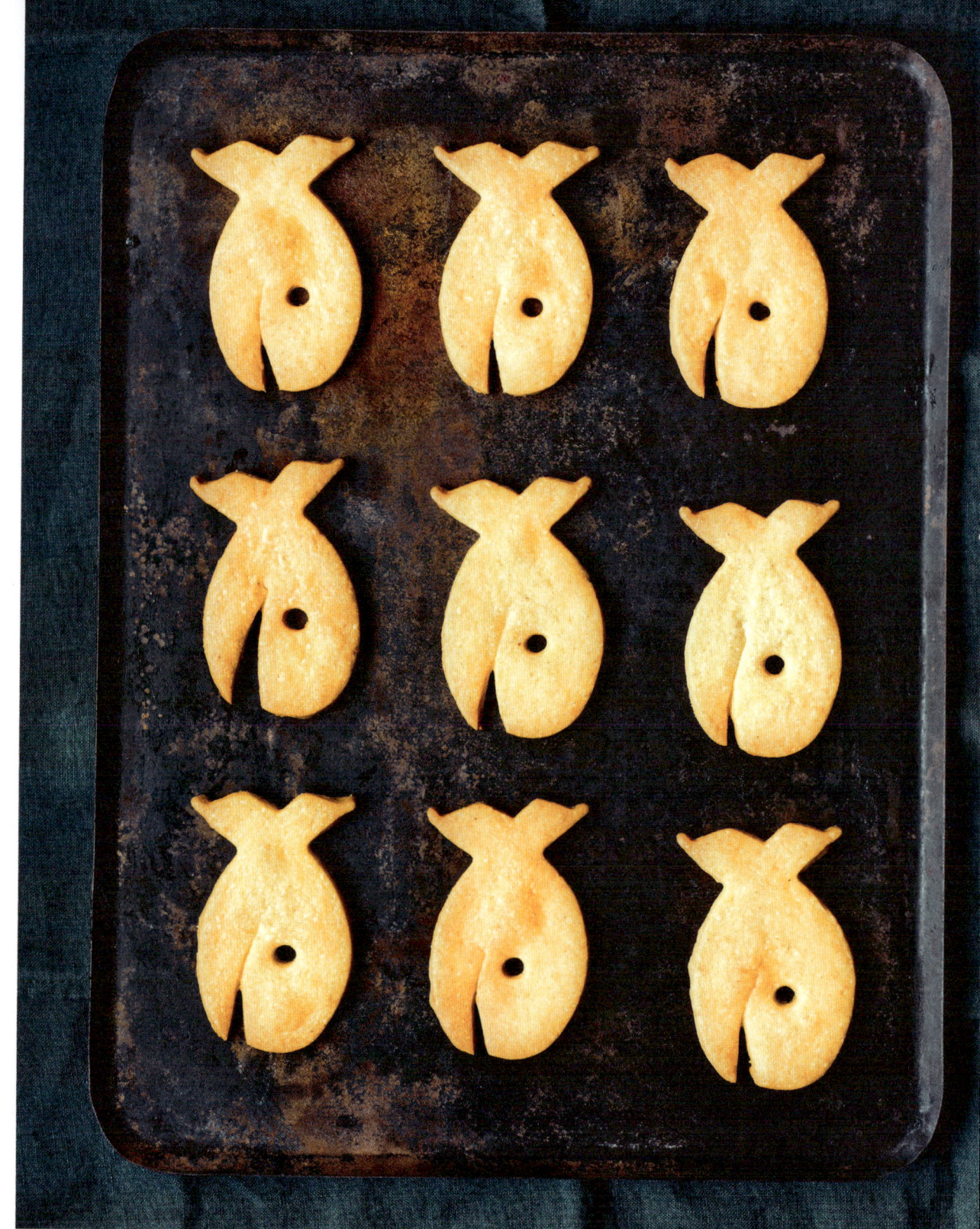

Cannabis Cheesy Goldfish Crackers

**MAKES ABOUT
24 CRACKERS**

These cheesy, buttery, smiling giant goldfish crackers are perfect for a special snack, since they are rich and addictively delicious for the cheese lover. If you spike them nicely with homemade Cannabutter (page 160), they may just give you amazing dreams, too! Be sure to try these infused crackers one bite at a time, until you know how potent they are. You can adjust the potency of your crackers by increasing or decreasing the proportion of cannabutter to butter. Remember that edibles can take up to three hours to exhibit their full effect.

The key to getting the goldfish shape is to augment a diamond ring cookie cutter (see Sources, page 178) by elongating the round portion, and adding a dent in the jewel part for the tail. To make the eye of the goldfish, just use a drinking straw once you have cut out the dough. Of course you may use any shape cookie cutter you choose. This recipe also works well using gluten-free flour. Enjoy responsibly!

8 ounces extra-sharp cheddar cheese, grated, at room temperature

7 ounces unsalted butter, at room temperature

1 ounce (2 tablespoons) Cannabutter (page 160), at room temperature

12 ounces (2⅓ cups) unbleached white all-purpose flour or gluten-free flour, plus more for dusting

1½ teaspoons fine sea salt

¼ teaspoon cayenne pepper

In a food processor, blend the cheese with the butter and cannabutter until creamy and uniform. You will likely have to scrape down the bowl a couple of times to achieve the right consistency. Alternatively, use a stand

CONTINUED

mixer with a paddle attachment. If you don't have a food processor or you'd like to get a bit of an arm workout, use a bowl and wooden mixing spoon instead. Make sure the cheese, butter, and cannabutter are at room temperature.

Add the flour, salt, and cayenne and mix, using low power pulses, until a dough forms. Turn out the dough onto plastic wrap, flatten into a disk, then wrap and chill in the fridge for about 1 hour.

Preheat the oven to 375°F. Line a large baking sheet with parchment paper.

Roll out the chilled dough just shy of ¼ inch thick on parchment paper, dusting with a little flour if necessary to prevent sticking.

Using a diamond-ring cookie cutter, cut out the fish shapes and place them on the prepared baking sheet. Then use a drinking straw to cut out an eye for each one and a sharp knife to cut a little smile.

Bake for 18 to 20 minutes, or until the crackers are beginning to brown on the edges. Remove the pan from the oven and transfer the crackers to a wire rack to cool. Store in an airtight container at room temperature for up to 1 week or in the freezer for up to 3 months.

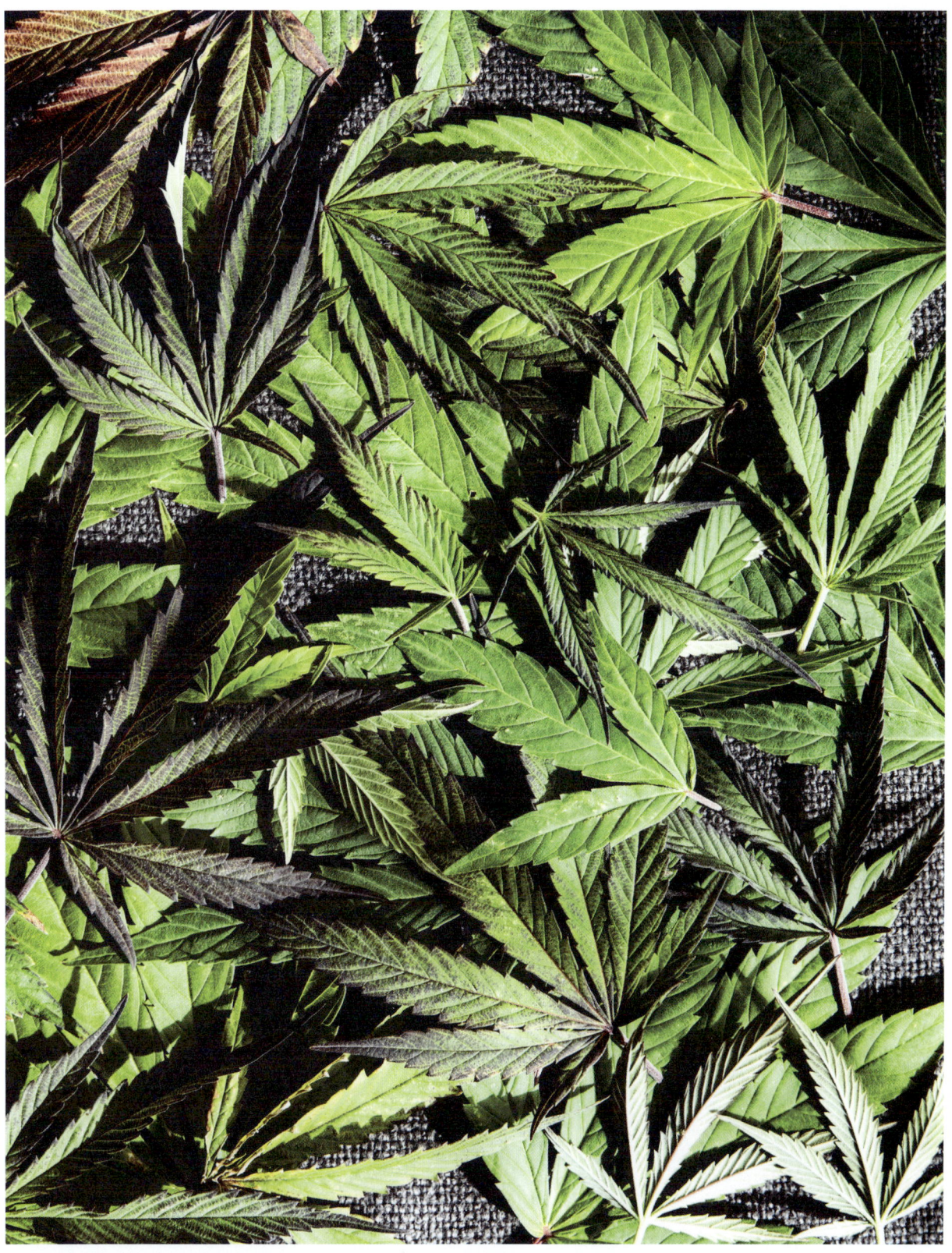

Infused Chocolate Shell

SERVES 8 TO 10

If you're a fan of chocolate-dipped ice cream cones, then this is the recipe for you. This infused chocolate shell offers a delicate crunch to coat ice cream in a cone or a cup. Another delicious option is to coat frozen banana chunks with it. This is a vegan recipe, relying on coconut oil and natural dairy-free dark chocolate. You control how potent this recipe is by altering the proportion of infused Cannaoil and coconut oil. I use refined virgin coconut oil in this recipe to keep the coconut flavor mild, but you may use any virgin coconut oil.

1 quart (or more) vanilla ice cream or dairy-free frozen dessert

6 ounces dark chocolate, chopped

1 ounce (2 tablespoons) Cannaoil (page 163)

1 ounce (2 tablespoons) coconut oil

Chopped nuts or sprinkles (optional)

Prescoop your ice cream into serving cups or cones, or impale each scoop with a Popsicle stick. Freeze until hard.

Just before serving, place the chocolate, cannaoil, and coconut oil in a 1- or 2-cup glass measuring cup. Heat in the microwave on high for 20 seconds on high. Stir to promote even melting. Continue to heat the mixture in the microwave in 10-second bursts, stirring between heating. When the mixture is just liquid, it's ready to pour over your ice cream or to dip your cones. Add the nuts or sprinkles, if using. The infused chocolate shell will harden into a delicious, thin layer that will shatter when you bite into it.

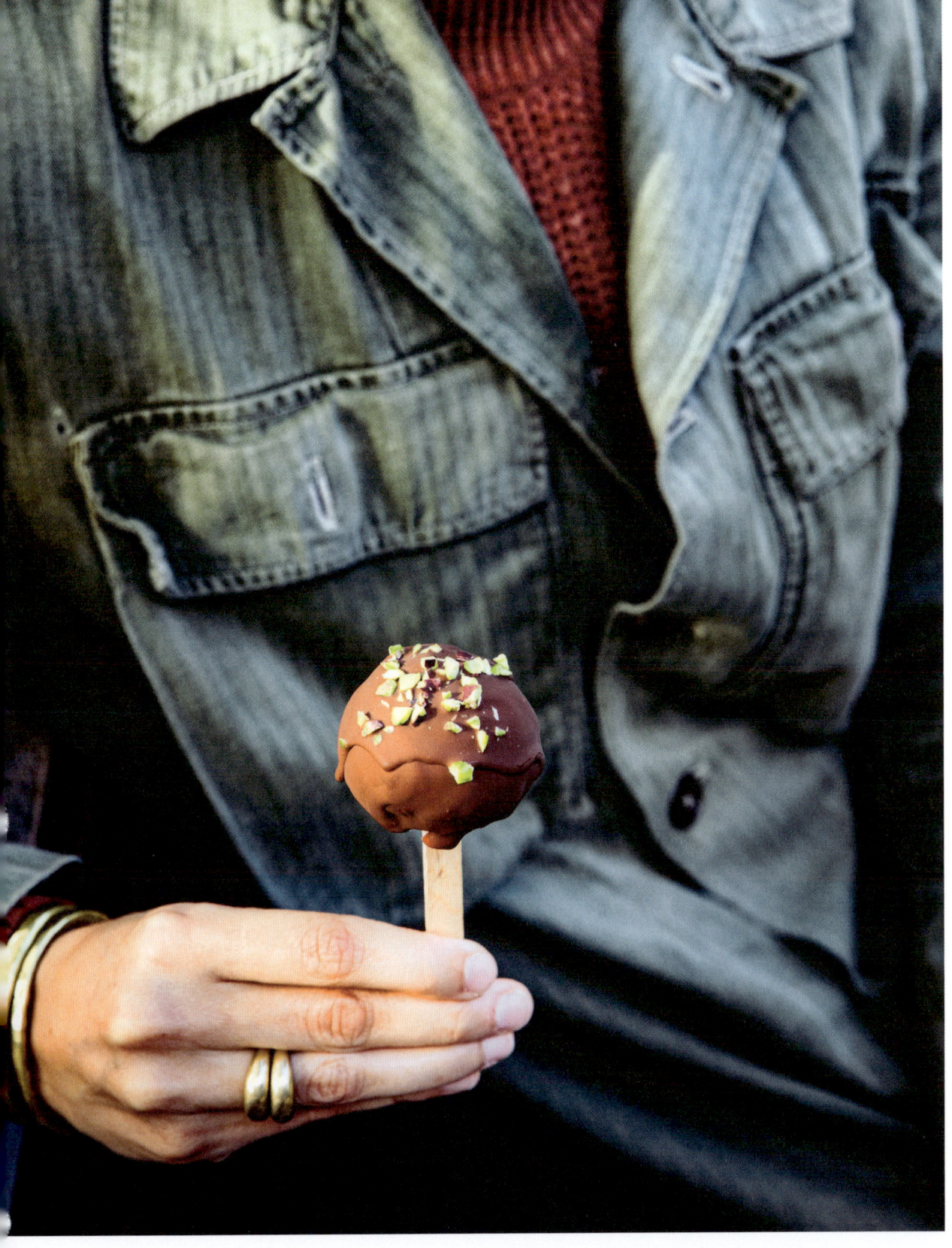

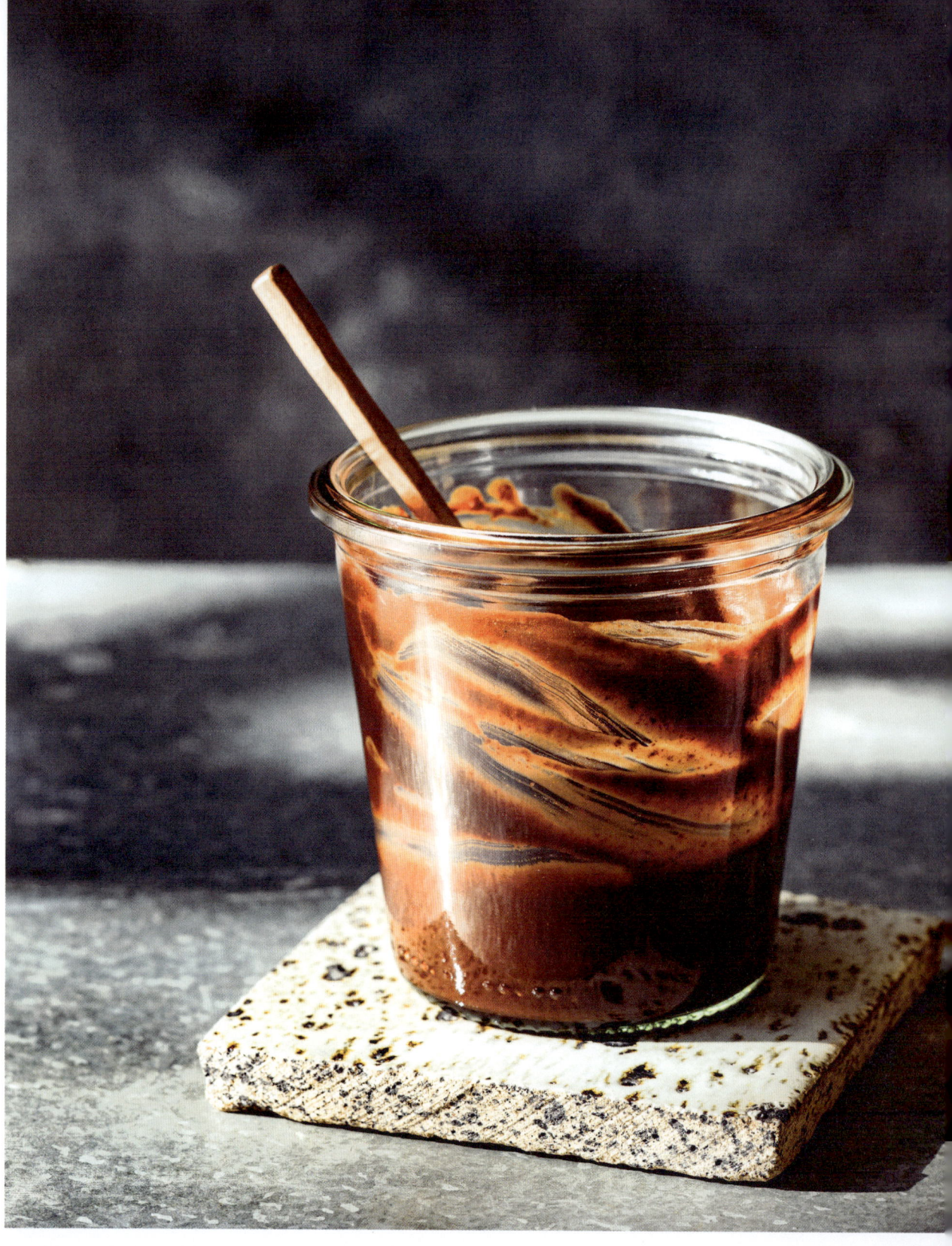

Infused Chocolate Sauce

MAKES APPROXIMATELY 1¼ CUPS

Here is my version of the perfect hot fudge sundae chocolate sauce. It's chocolatey, smooth, and unctuous, without being too sweet. It also happens to be a very simple and frugal recipe that you can make and use in under an hour. Just measure, mix, boil—and snap! The effect of this sauce depends on the amount and potency of your Cannabutter or Cannaoil. You may adjust the proportion of butter to Cannabutter to impact the level of cannabinoids in your sauce.

⅔ cup water

4 ounces unsweetened chocolate, chopped

1 cup granulated sugar

1 ounce butter or coconut oil

1 ounce (2 tablespoons) Cannabutter or Cannaoil (page 160)

¼ teaspoon sea salt

½ teaspoon pure vanilla extract

In a medium saucepan, combine the water, chocolate, sugar, butter, cannabutter, and salt. Place on medium-high heat and bring to a boil, stirring with a whisk. Simmer until the sauce begins to thicken a bit. Remove from the heat and stir in the vanilla extract, whisking until smooth. Cool until warm, then blend for a few seconds using an immersion blender or a regular blender (this creates a smooth, velvety texture). Pour over ice cream or non-dairy frozen dessert for a fabulous sundae. Toasted nuts and whipped cream add the perfect final touches. Store in an airtight container in the fridge for up to 1 month.

Cannabis Tisane

One of the best perks of growing cannabis in your own garden is that you have access to the fresh leaves throughout much of the growing season. While these leaves have lower concentrations of cannabinoids and terpenes than you'll find in the bud, they contain just enough to soothe the mind and body. Since the small amount of THC present in these leaves is in the natural acid form, it won't get you high. These tisanes work well with either fresh or dried cannabis leaves. Choose healthy leaves no more than 3 inches in diameter for tisanes. You'll find these small tender leaves have the best flavor and provide a mellow impact on the body.

The mint and lemon verbena variations are especially good during the day and just as delicious served warm or cold. And for a luxe evening tisane, add fresh or dried lavender to the pot.

Quick-dried cannabis leaves

To quick-dry the cannabis, preheat oven to 170°F. Spread small leaves in a shallow layer on a baking sheet. Bake until the leaves are crisp dry, about 15 minutes. Begin checking for doneness after 10 minutes in the oven. The leaves should not brown, but will be stiff and snap easily when they are fully dried. Cool and store airtight in a cool dark spot for up to a year.

Frozen cannabis bud and leaves

To freeze freshly picked cannabis bud and leaves, simply place them in a single layer on a baking sheet. Freeze until firm, then store frozen bud and leaves airtight in the freezer. They will remain frozen and usable for several years.

CONTINUED

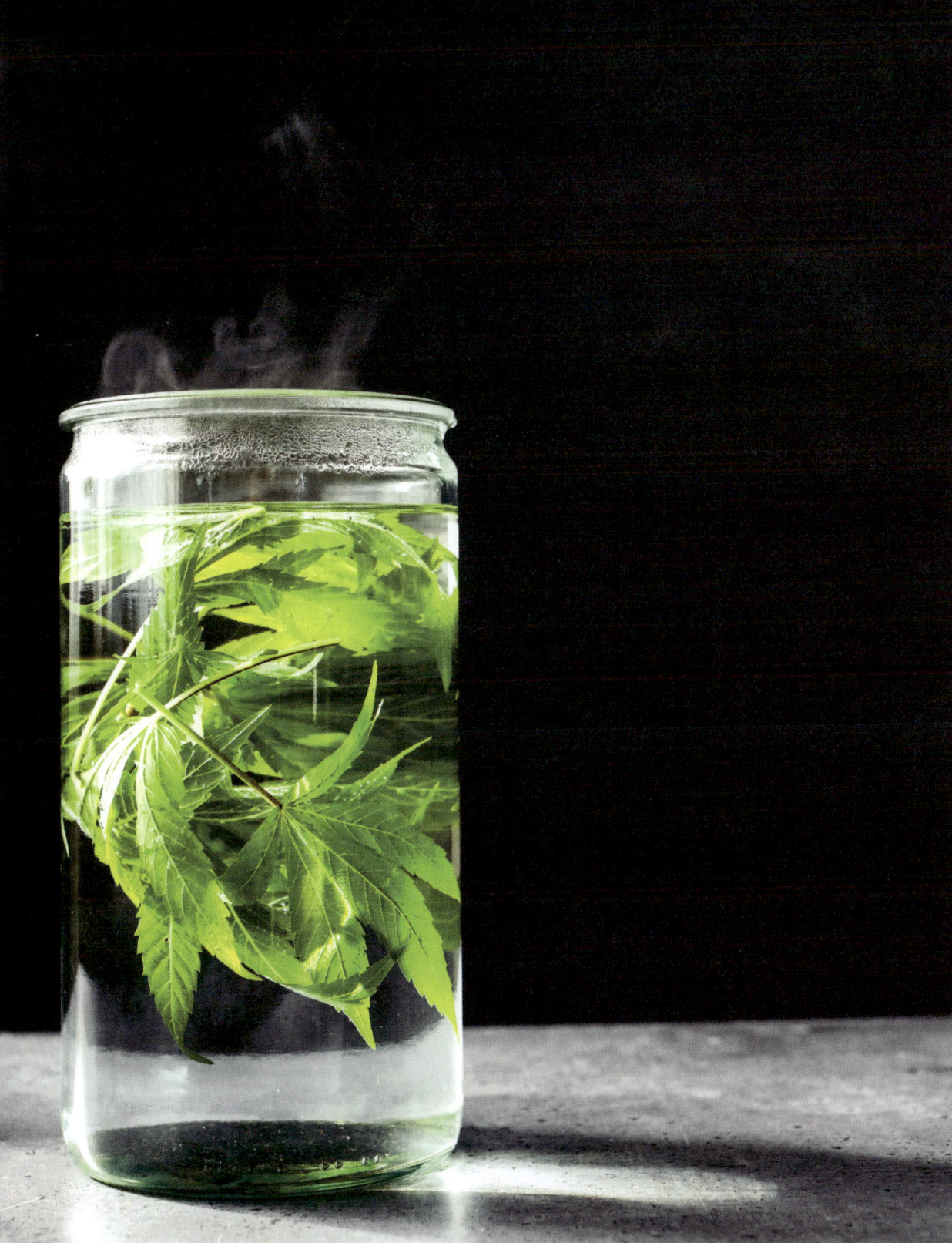

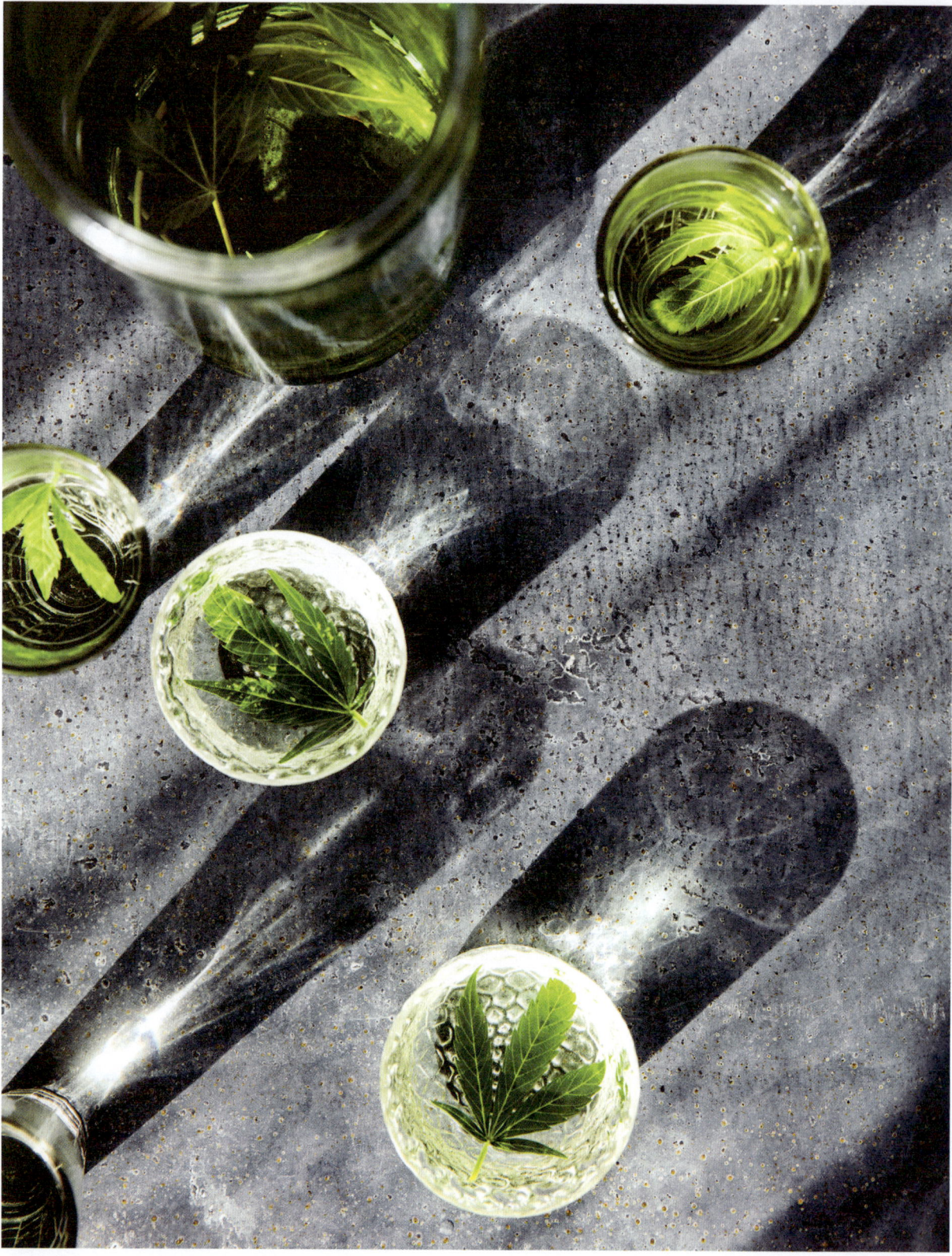

SERVES 4 TO 6

Cannabis Tisane

½ cup fresh, frozen, or dried
small cannabis leaves

Place the cannabis leaves in a large preheated teapot. Pour boiling water over the leaves and allow to steep for 4 minutes. Strain into teacups and enjoy.

For iced cannabis tisane, strain the hot tisane into an ice-filled carafe.

VARIATIONS

CANNAMINT TISANE
Uplifting and bright

Add ¼ cup fresh mint leaves to the teapot before steeping. Dried mint may also be used if fresh is not available.

LEMON VERBENA AND CANNABIS TISANE
Delicious and invigorating

Add ¼ cup fresh lemon verbena leaves to the teapot before steeping. This is excellent iced, served with a squeeze of fresh lemon.

Note: For a hit of summer freshness in the off-season, I freeze lemon verbena leaves and cannabis budlets when they are available—then use them in tisanes throughout the year.

LAVENDER AND CANNABIS TISANE
Soothing and warming to help you drift off to sleep

Add 2 teaspoons fresh or dried lavender blossoms to the teapot before steeping.

Glossary

adventitious roots. Roots that form from a non-root plant part, such as a stem. Adventitious roots are distinct from the taproot.

anaerobic. Natural biochemical processes that use no oxygen.

anandamide. The name, from a Sanskrit word meaning "bliss," given to N-arachidonoylethanolamine (AEA), a potent cannabinoid that is made in the human body. Discovered and named by Raphael Mechoulam with William A. Devane and Lumír Hanuš in 1992.

auto-flowers. Modern, non-photoperiod cannabis cultivars bred to begin flowering based on the age of the plant rather than seasonal changes in day/night periods.

clone. As used in this book, a clone refers to a rooted cutting of a cannabis plant.

cola. A dense cluster of many small flowers growing in a group.

cotyledon. The embryonic leaves that emerge from the sprouted seed. Cotyledons are also called seed leaves and serve to nourish the baby plant while it produces its first set of true leaves. Cannabis plants have two cotyledons and are thus dicots.

day-neutral. Plants that are not dependent on the seasonal day/night light fluctuations to trigger blooming.

decarboxylated. A chemical that has lost its carboxyl group (a molecule composed of one carbon atom, two oxygen atoms, and one hydrogen atom). Decarboxylation of the cannabinoids in cannabis bud occurs with the addition of heat, oxygen, light, and time.

dioecious. A plant that has male and female flowers on separate plants, thus creating male and female plants.

endocannabinoid. A compound created by the human body to modulate the endocannabinoid system. Two endocannabinoids so far discovered are anandamide and 2-AG.

entourage effect. The whole impact of cannabinoids and terpenes on the body and mind of the consumer. This term was coined by Raphael Mechoulam and Shimon Ben-Shabat as a way of describing their observations about the varying impact of cannabis on people.

F1 generation. The phenotypes expressed by the first generation of a plant cross-fertilization.

F2 generation. The phenotypes expressed by the second generation of a plant cross.

foliar feed. The act of spraying a substance on plant leaves to give them a boost of nutrients. Compost tea is a commonly used as a foliar feed. The plant's leaves benefit from the micro-nutrients and helpful microbes in the foliar feed.

hardening off. The act of exposing tender, new young or potted plants to current outdoor garden conditions, such as bright sun, temperature swings, and moisture fluctuations in order to prepare them for planting outside.

hemp. US law defines hemp as *C. sativa* containing 0.3 percent or less of THC after harvest. Traditionally, hemp was defined as those cannabis plants grown and harvested for fiber.

homeostasis. Derived from the Greek *homeo* (like) and *stasis* (state of being), the process by which any living thing creates stable physiological processes to foster health for itself.

inflorescence. The entire flowering structure of the plant, including the flowers, bracts, stems, and stalks.

internode. The distance on the cannabis stem between nodes of emergent leaves and/or lateral stems. Long internodes are common on hemp.

monoecious. A plant that has male and female flowers on the same plant, or a plant whose flowers are perfect (each flower has both male and female parts).

mycorrhizae. The very slender filaments of soil fungus that permeate healthy garden soil.

nug. Slang for cannabis flower clusters, either fresh on the plant or dried; bud.

photoperiod sensitive. Describes plants that rely on the seasonal day/night light fluctuations to trigger blooming. All cannabis is photoperiod sensitive except *Cannabis ruderalis* and modern hybrids known as auto-flowers.

phytocannabinoid. A compound created by a plant that modulates the endocannabinoid system. Cannabis has hundreds of unique phytocannabinoids, including THC and CBD.

psychedelic. A substance that creates a state of euphoria or distortions in perception or an altered awareness. THC is the cannabinoid that is chiefly responsible for the psychedelic effects felt after consuming cannabis products.

psychoactive. A substance that impacts the mental processes without creating a psychedelic experience. CBD and many cannabinoids are psychoactive but not psychedelic.

schedule 1 drug. Cannabis is listed in schedule 1 in the Controlled Substances Act, administered by the US Drug Enforcement Administration.

strain. The term used to describe a specific named type of cannabis, i.e., Blue Dream is a strain of cannabis. The term *strain* is increasingly being replaced by the more horticulturally appropriate term *cultivar*.

sugar leaves. The tiny, sticky leaves that grow in the large clusters of cannabis flowers. They are so named because of their sugary, white appearance at the end of the growing season.

terpenes. A large group of molecules made by many plants, including cannabis. Terpenes are volatile organic compounds that are very fragrant and have diverse physiological impacts on the body, especially when consumed with cannabinoids. Terpenes abundant in cannabis include limonene, pinene, myrcene, linalool, caryophyllene, and geraniol.

tincture. A solution of cannabis and alcohol. Tinctures are a traditional method of consuming cannabis.

tisane. A beverage made by soaking plant material in hot water, also known as herbal tea. Connoisseurs typically only use the word *tea* to refer to a decoction of tea leaves (*Camellia sinensis*) in hot water.

tissue culture. A method of producing a new genetically complete plant by growing a tiny part of a living plant on a specialized growth medium in a laboratory setting. Tissue culture plants—true clones—are different from the rooted cuttings typically referred to as clones by many cannabis growers.

trichomes. Tiny structures that emerge from the epidermis of plants and create and hold resins. Trichomes are usually found in greatest density on flower buds and the small leaves that surround them. There are a few different types of trichomes, but all of them are tiny, sticky with resin, and found on the outer surfaces of the plant.

Sources

Cannabis seeds

Dispensary: If you live in a state where cannabis is legal, a dispensary is a great place to purchase cannabis seeds. Ask your budtender about both the grower and the breeder of the seeds to understand what to expect from your seeds. Cannabis seed breeding programs are just starting to create garden worthy, high quality cannabis. Humboldt Seed Company is a well-regarded breeder of cannabis seeds for the USA.

Online: Because cannabis is not federally legal in the USA, most online cannabis seed sellers are located in Europe.

Sensi Seeds: *www.sensiseeds.com/en*
DNA Genetics: *www.dnagenetics.com*
Dinafem: *www.dinafem.org/en*

Trade: Befriend fellow cannabis gardeners in your community and start a cannabis seed exchange.

Diamond ring cookie cutter
Used to make the Cannabis Cheesy Goldfish Crackers (see page 165)

www.annclarkcookiecutters.com/product/diamond-ring-cookie-cutter/best-sellers

E. B. Stone Recipe 420 Potting Soil
Available at your local nursery

www.ebstone.org

Felco pruners
www.felco.com

Flower Power planting mix
American Soil & Stone (for San Francisco Bay Area residents)

www.americansoil.com

Grove Bags
Cannabis storage bags

www.grovebags.com

Hida Tool
Excellent selection of Japanese gardening tools

www.hidatool.com

MightyCrop
Plant-staking system

www.mightycrop.com

Phylos Bioscience
Cannabis plant sex testing

www.phylos.bio

Source Turbo
Tabletop extractor

www.extractcraft.com/shop/source-turbo

Steep Hill
Cannabis potency testing

www.steephill.com

For an up-to-date bibliography, see www.pennybarthel.com

Acknowledgments

Thank you to John Barthel, my husband. Your constant love and support are life-giving. Plus, you are my favorite cannabis-concoction beta tester.

Thank you to my children, Calvin Barthel and Lucy Barthel, for letting me go from hard-ass mom of your teen selves to a cannabis nerd. I love you two so much.

Thank you to Jane Purinton, Paige Baumgartner, and John Purinton for cheering me on in my cannabis journey, and to John Spencer and Sally Stempler for your enthusiastic support.

Let's Sesh Workshops partners Kaisha-Dyan McMillan and Deirdre Greene are two other legs on my three-legged cannabis stool. I appreciate all the amazing students at our Let's Sesh Workshops. We've grown together as cannabis nerds!

To my Ladies Group, you listened, trusting me even when it felt a little scary to be talking about weed: Kate Rankin, Julia Bailey, Mae Chan, Kim Howard, Raquel Van Noord, Beth Thomsen, and Janis Connallon. Special thanks to Mae for wisely coaching me about business avatars, and to Julia for strategic wordsmithing.

Thank you to my weekly Bible study small group for your support, and for learning with me on this cannabis journey as we all went from prohibition to the present: Kim Howard, Jonathan Howard, Brian Conery, Janet Conery, John Barthel, Pete Docter, and Amanda Docter.

To the folks in my book groups, thank you for showing me the importance of reading and growing from books, and for taking me seriously when I said, "I'm writing a book." To those not already mentioned: Kathie Johnson, Susan Phillips, Chris Anderson, Laura Sera, Carol Aust, Christina Robinson, Liz Sutton, Carrie Salazar, Bernadette Powell, Laura Allen, Carla Golden, Joyce McCallister, Angie Woolman, Tom Schuetz, Mark Westover, and Jackie Ato.

Thank you to the Hipline community, especially Samar Nassar and Gabriela Nassar Covareli for lavish encouragement, Hana Raja for great feedback, Aya Brackett, Ali Lawrence, and so many other amazing women! Special thanks to Karina Schuetz for constant encouragement in my day-to-day reality of writing while extroverted.

Shout out to Oaksterdam for teaching me about cannabis horticulture.

Props to the Ten Speed/Random House team who made this book a reality: Kim Keller, Lisa Bieser, and Dan Myers, and to Andrea Portanova and Natalie Yera for promoting the book and getting the word out. And thanks to copyeditor Dolores York and proofreader Kathy Brock.

Thank you to Erin Scott, Lillian Kang, and Nicola Parisi for your stunning photography—you brought this book to life!

Thank you to my agent Amy Collins of Squid Ink Literary Agency for moving this book from my head into reality.

Leslie Bennett: Thank you for saying, "You could write a book."

Stefani Bittner: Thank you for saying, "Write this book and I'll be the first to buy it."

Kaisha-Dyan McMillan: Thank you for telling me that I was going to be the Martha Stewart of weed someday—and for so much more.

Johanna Silver: Thank you for sharing a passion for gardening and seeing something special in me.

Angie Nierva, Nevin Berger, Amy St. George, John Alexander, and my fellow local cannabis gardeners: Thanks for growing cannabis plants outside in the garden, where they belong.

Thanks to Drew Farwell, Kate Gaudette, Ryan Carnavale, Jamie Baumgartner, Susan Marks, and Dan Grace for sharing cannabis wisdom so generously.

And thanks to Ripe band members for showing me how to roll a perfect joint via FaceTime, while you were in the green room, just about to go on stage: Robbie, Calvin, Josh, Tory, Nadav, John, and Sampson.

Index

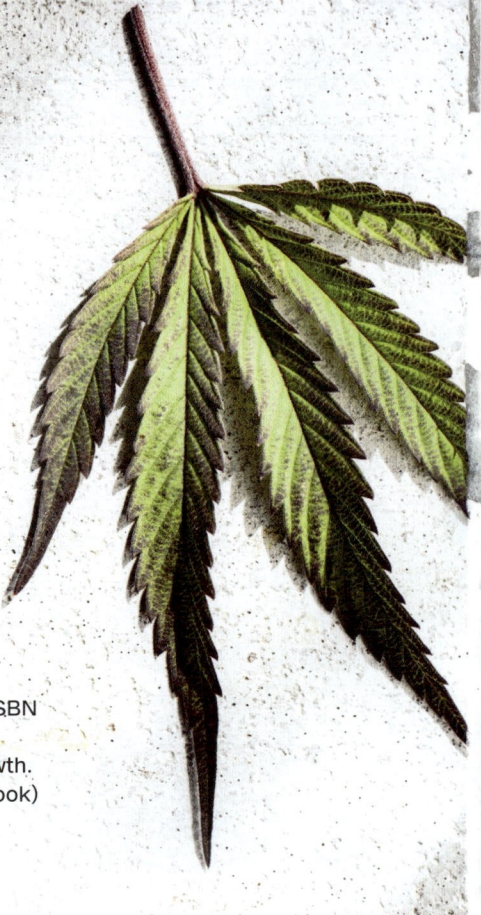

Published in the United States by Ten Speed Press, an imprint of
Random House, a division of Penguin Random House LLC, New York.
www.tenspeed.com

Ten Speed Press and the Ten Speed Press colophon are registered
trademarks of Penguin Random House LLC.

Library of Congress Cataloging-in-Publication Data
    Names: Barthel, Penny, 1965– author.
    Title: The cannabis gardener : a beginner's guide to growing vibrant,
        healthy plants in every region / Penny Barthel.
    Description: First edition. | [Emeryville], California : Ten Speed Press,
        [2121] | Includes bibliographical references and index.
    Identifiers: LCCN 2020020080 (print) | LCCN 2020020081 (ebook) | ISBN
        9781984858849 (hardcover) | ISBN 9781984858856 (ebook)
    Subjects: LCSH: Cannabis. | Gardening. | Cannabis—Seedlings—Growth.
    Classification: LCC SB295.C35 B37 2021 (print) | LCC SB295.C35 (ebook)
        | DDC 633.7/9—dc23
    LC record available at https://lccn.loc.gov/2020020080
    LC ebook record available at https://lccn.loc.gov/2020020081

Hardcover ISBN: 978-1-9848-5884-9
eBook ISBN: 978-1-9848-5885-6

Printed in China

Editor: Kim Keller
Designer: Lisa Schneller Bieser
Art director: Emma Campion
Production designer: Mari Gill
Production manager: Dan Myers
Food & botanicals stylist: Lillian Kang
Prop stylist: Erin Scott
Photo assistant and model: Nicola Parisi
Copyeditor: Dolores York
Proofreader: Kathy Brock
Indexer: Ken DellaPenta
Publicist: Natalie Yera
Marketer: Andrea Portanova

10 9 8 7 6 5 4 3 2 1

First Edition

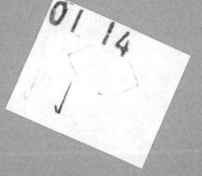